Divine Dining

365 Devotions to Guide You to Healthier Weight and Abundant Wellness

By Janet K. Brown

P
Pen-L Publishing
Fayetteville, Arkasnas
Pen-L.com

Divine Dining: 365 Devotions to Guide You to
Healthier Weight and Abundant Wellness

First Edition
ISBN: 978-0-9851274-3-5

All scripture is KJV unless otherwise noted.

I am super liking *Divine Dining*. It is a wonderful book. Speaks daily to me. Thank you for writing your story, sharing it with all of us. – Bonnie Lanthripe, Oklahoma City, OK

Wow! Am I having a feast! A feast of inspiration and revelation after reading your book, *Divine Dining.*
– Madeleine Calcott, Australia

Over the years, I have watched Janet Brown practice what she teaches. The emotional healing she received from the Lord triggered her own weight loss. Because of this healing, she has been willing and able to reach out to other women struggling with the same issues. I have witnessed how her teachings, blog writings, and devotions are turning hearts toward God and changing lives through emotional healing.
– Debra Calloway

Divine Dining, was a great encouragement to me . . . . I have struggled with weight loss issues most of my adult life. As I read each entry, I realized I had not made God my partner in my attempt to lose weight and adopt a different attitude about the priority of food in my day to day living. I am looking forward to using this devotional each morning to assist me in adapting a life style that gives glory to God. – Sue Watson

Thank you for writing such an amazing devotional that talks about your struggles but also about your faith. I'm thankful I'm not alone in my journey to be a better me!!
–Rodney Brumbelow

I have struggled with my weight as long as I can remember. Finally there is a devotional that is directed at the core of my issue with obesity. One that is not another "diet" for me to follow until I "fall off the wagon again." I am so thankful I was able to get this book and be able to include it in my daily life changes to a healthier me, both physically and spiritually.
–Page2Page, Amazon

Also by Janet K. Brown

Victoria and the Ghost

Worth Her Weight

This book is dedicated to the thousands of men and women who strive to be Christians, but suffer from compulsive overeating they can't control.
THERE IS HOPE.

Introduction

My first diet started at age fourteen. Through marriage and the birth of three daughters, I gained more weight and suffered more emotional scarring. My health deteriorated physically and mentally. I reached two hundred fifty pounds. By then I was a wreck, with thoughts of suicide. Food dominated everything I did.

Our praise and worship leader at church began Christian Weight Controllers. He taught from his own battles, so he had no established curriculum, but it was God's blessing for me.

Over a period of two years, I lost ninety-five pounds. My mentor moved on and bequeathed the class to me. I taught it for several years, writing my own curriculum as I went. During that time, help also came in the form of a series of twelve-step programs. I have maintained my loss for seventeen years, but rarely teach, preferring instead to encourage on-on-one.

One tool in my recovery remains the daily reading of inspirational books. I found my library incomplete when I searched for one that combined a twelve-step program with God as the Higher Power. One night, God woke me in the middle of the night and gave me fourteen devotions that became the first of the three hundred and sixty-five in this book. The biggest secret to my success is giving up *my* will and letting God do it through me.

This book of daily devotions comes from my journals and memories. This is one woman's road for success. I pray these thoughts help others reach the same healing God gave to me. It's all about God.

Janet K. Brown

Divine
Dining

January 1

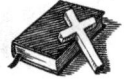

Repairer of Broken Walls

The Lord will guide you always; he will satisfy your needs in a sun-scorched land . . . you will be called Repairer of Broken Walls, Restorer of Streets with Dwellings. Isaiah 58: 11,12

Do you have moments when you feel like you're losing your mind? The definition of insanity is doing the same thing over and over and expecting different results. Sound familiar?

A psychiatrist once told me trying to willingly destroy one's self is not sane. Compulsive overeaters kill themselves slowly with legal means, but it's no less crazy.

Resentment, envy, and anger tear down the mind's protective walls. The enemy of the soul can oppress an unguarded mind.

In my case, these emotions created havoc and caused emotional imbalance; insanity, if you will.

Of my own free will, I chose to ignore the enemy's influence and gave my mind and my body to the Lord's control. God used my day-to-day actions to repair those walls and restore in me normality.

Healing is contingent on spiritual condition.

Prayer: Lord, today take my thoughts, my will, and my choices and let them be Yours.

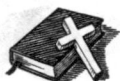

January 2

Stiff-Necked, Unrelenting Will

. . . let the Lord go with us. Although this is a stiff-necked people, forgive our wickedness and our sin, and take us as your inheritance. Exodus 34:9

We read about the stiff-necked will of the Israelites. God provided for their needs, but still they complained and wanted more.

How many times have I gone against everything I thought I wanted, everything that my family, my work, my Christian walk demanded so that I could "control" my situation.

Friends and family advised me to use will power and refrain from overeating. The truth was I had an unrelenting will I use every day.

My will power overcame every rational thought to say, "I will to eat what I like, and I won't be controlled by anyone else in choosing what I eat." The craziness of this principle was that my will power overcame my conscious goals and desires. Like turning on a tank of oxygen near the fireplace, my invincible will power/won't power consumed my sanity and my life.

No power but God's power is strong enough to overcome a stiff-necked rebellion. Are you a control freak? Has it ruined everything you hold dear?

Prayer: Lord, help me to release my stiff-necked will power unto You.

January 3

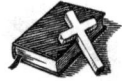

Desires of Your Heart

Delight yourself in the Lord and he will give you the desire of your heart. Commit your way to the Lord; trust in him, and he will do this: Psalms 37:4-5 NIV

God loves His children.

You are one of His children.

He wants to give you the desire of your heart.

Is your desire to have your compulsion not control you? God is stronger, His ways more sure than you can imagine.

Here's an actual example of how God helped me one morning:

I planned to stop by the donut shop on my way to work the next morning. I arose, rushed my preparation, and left early to have time for the extra errand.

But God's ways are infinitely stronger, more sure than mine. According to the habit I'd established, I prayed during my quiet time that God's will, not mine, be done. God heard and answered that request.

When I came close to the donut shop, I had this over-whelming desire to not feel stuffed since I had so much work to do. Where did I get that thought? It hadn't been there when I left the house. I arrived at my job astounded that I had failed to complete my mission to buy donuts.

God wants to give you the desire of your heart, but you must ask it of Him and then leave it in His hands to fix.

Prayer: Lord, I truly want Your will today. Let it be.

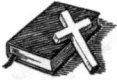

January 4

Weary In Well Doing

Let us not become weary in doing good, for at the proper time we will reap a harvest if we do not give up. Galatians 6:9 NIV

Martyrs for Christ existed in the past and they still do in modern days. I'm not one of them, but sometimes I think I am.

We work hard doing things around the church. That's good, but is it what God wants?

An example tells my experience. Others may relate.

I do whatever is asked of me in church. I see others lauded for their work, but not me. Resentment springs up in my mind, poisoning my system until I'm physically ill. My body grows weary and susceptible to virus and infections.

I say, "God, I'm doing everything for You."

God says, "What have you done for Me? I asked you to spend time talking with Me this morning, but you couldn't since there was a church meeting at nine. I asked you to eat nutritiously so you would have more energy at the end of the day for your family, but you didn't. Instead, you made a cake for the class social and ate it. Because of that, you had to make another one to take in place of the first cake.

God tells us not to be weary. When we do something at church that He asks us to do, He will give supernatural strength, but first, be sure it's what He asks of you.

Prayer: Lord, like Mary, who sat at Jesus' feet, let me today choose the best part.

January 5

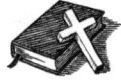

My Self-esteem is Dragging

For we are God's workmanship, created in Christ Jesus to do good works, which God prepared in advance for us to do.
Ephesians 2:10 NIV

Compulsive overeating is a symptom of something wrong. As a rule, when we suffer low self-esteem, the extra weight we gain magnifies the problem. When we overeat, our esteem plummets. Common sense tells us that if we do what we like, we'll be happy. Instead, we sink lower into depression. Many of us excel at a host of challenges, but fail in how we eat. Then we accept failure as the theme of our lives.

I've lived for Christ since I gave my heart to Him in vacation Bible school when I was seven. I drifted, but came back to God while in college. I read verses like the one above and implemented self talk about being a creation of, and an example of, God's workmanship. There was always a but. But *I* don't follow Christ like I should. But *I* don't have enough faith.

Now I experience a miracle from Christ when I relinquish control to Him and give up the fight. He completes me. He adorns my days with peace. He gives me worth.

I used to be able to list ten things I hated about myself, but it took God's power to come up with a list of ten things I liked about myself. Now I can. Can you?

Prayer: Lord, take control of me. In doing so, You make me worthy.

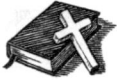

January 6

It's Just Food

Their destiny is destruction, their god is their stomach, and their glory is in their shame. Their mind is on earthly things.
Philippians 3:19 NIV

Does this internal monologue sound familiar? "It's just food, not a serious problem. Everyone has to eat. It's not like being an alcoholic or a drug addict."

Our families reinforce that thought by saying we just need to cut back on food. Good Christian friends laugh about diving into that cake brought by Sister so-and-so. Friends giggle about starting their diets tomorrow. Every magazine and TV station offers the latest fad in weight loss.

To a compulsive overeater, this isn't funny. Compulsion in any form will destroy our bodies and our minds.

One night, my daughter phoned me. A thief had forced open her back door. She feared the intruder was still inside. She had called the police, but wanted a loved one with her. I told her I would come, but my food compulsion stopped me. I had binged on candy and muffins and lay in my recliner listless and nauseous. If her husband hadn't called, I might have left her alone. I would have hated myself for it, but the food had overcome my ability to function.

Has food ever immobilized you? Has it made you yell at your kids or your husband? Have you turned down a chance to work for the Lord because of how you felt or because it cut into mealtime? Is the problem "just food?"

Prayer: Lord, heal my compulsion. Allow me to be used according to Your will.

January 7

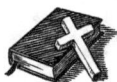

The Protection of the Wren Cactus

To him who is able to keep you from falling and to present you before his glorious presence without fault and with great joy. Jude 24 NIV

If food compulsion is part of our carnal life, danger lurks whenever we leave God's protection.

At a friend's country home, we noticed a cactus bush three to four feet high with a nest of wrens on one side. We commented.

"That's our wren cactus, our sanctuary for birds," our friend told us.

On the other side of the bush, we spotted baby mocking-birds. Instead of flying to high places to be safe from the coyotes and deer, birds make their home here in a small bush. On examination, we noticed birds fly into the cactus without touching the prickly thorns. A larger animal would be unable to do that, so the birds make their nests in perfect safety right under the noses of their enemies.

God is our wren cactus. He protects us from certain defeat and destruction while in the presence of food that would tempt us. His loving arms encircle us. The enemy can't get past His defense.

Prayer: When I'm at a restaurant or party, a potluck, or another's home, I'm vulnerable without your hedge. Please protect me today, Lord.

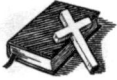

January 8

Are You a Sinner?

If we claim we have not sinned, we make him out to be a liar, and his word has no place in our lives. 1 John 1:10 NIV

Look at your life. Have you given your heart to Jesus? I did at age seven in a vacation Bible school.

Have you lived a consistent Christian life, or was there a time when you strayed from God? After high school graduation, I rebelled. I came back to the Lord in college.

Do you attend church? Have you worked for Christ? Do you resent being called a sinner? I did. My only discredit was over-eating. During my thirties and forties, I prayed for the Lord to help me lose weight, but every time I stopped a diet, I gained more.

Have you faced your gluttony and admitted rebellion? That's what I did.

We are powerless to control our innate sinful nature. Only Jesus can save. Jesus can only take those sins that we release to Him. We hold out our problem with food for the Lord to see and touch, but we fail to put it into His hands and leave it there.

Think about your food compulsion. Does it cause other sins such as dishonesty or resentment, even anger? We might start with the sin of gluttony but add to it a myriad of other sins. They sap our desire to live for God. Without God, we face defeat.

Prayer: I give up, Lord. I need Your forgiveness and your strength to overcome my petty rebellion. This time, I lay it in Your hands.

January 9

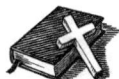

Take My Life, My Will, My Choices Today

*Not that we are competent in ourselves to claim anything for
ourselves, but our competence comes from God.*
2 Corinthians 3:5

We go to our place of worship and pray, "Lord, help me stay
on my diet and lose weight. Help me lose my cravings." When
we walk away, we feel shame. That's too trivial a plea for God.
He wouldn't answer a prayer like that.

However, when our children call and ask us to pray, nothing
is too small. Are we more loving than God? He wants to hear
about anything that affects His children.

Do we stay on our diets for days? A month? Three? With
only our will power, we can last for a period of time, but, without Christ changing us, eventually, compulsions win. Carnal
desire overwhelms. A gallon of ice cream calls our name.

We can identify with Paul's prayer. "Lord, that which I
desire to do, I don't, and that which I want to stop, I do."

We might add, "Despite effort, sacrifice, and nutritional
education, I remain powerless, with my life unmanageable. I
give it to You. Though it's not much, here it is."

When we pray that way and mean it, what a surprise.
Everything changes. God moves.

After walking the path with Christ, we can spot the difference when we forget and take the reins of our life once more.
Disaster follows the wake of an emotional tornado, and we
know what must be done.

We pray every morning "take my will, my life, and my
choices this day." Then, put the steering wheel in His hands.

My control = disaster   God's control = power

Prayer: Lord, take my life, my will, my choices today.

9

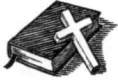

January 10

Why Doesn't God Help Every Time?

Let us hold unswervingly to the hope we profess, for he who promised is faithful. Hebrews 10:23 NIV

Have your prayers been answered by God? Have you experienced His move on your behalf to solve a problem?

Personal experience #1

I craved one of my binge foods. I prayed but still went to the store to buy my drug of choice. Before I found it, I ran into a friend or found something else that engaged my interest. I walked out of the store without my treat. I never made a conscious choice to not buy the food, but God's will was done in my life because I prayed. The experience causes tingles even now.

Personal experience #2

I prayed, went to the store and bought the food. I then binged all afternoon.

What's the difference? Our spiritual condition.

Abstinence is dependent on OUR dependence on God. We can say the words, but God knows if it comes from the heart.

Think about it next time. Did you leave it in His hands or did you pick it back up after prayer? Relying on self doesn't work. Relying on God works every time.

Prayer: Lord, teach me to depend on You as a toddler relies on his parent.

January 11

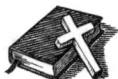

Poor Me

. . . for it is God who works in you, to will and to act according to his good purpose. Do everything without complaining or arguing . . . Philippians 2:13, 14

God gives you victory over temptation. He takes over your life and leads in a different direction. The weight lifts. Your self-esteem escalates.

Do you say, "I wish I had something sweet. I wish I could go to the restaurant and pick what I really want. I never get to relax and eat the good stuff."

Are you ducking your head? I am. After God works miracles for us, we throw ourselves a pity party. We should kneel and repent. God calls us to His good purpose. Our job is to cease complaining or arguing. God requires a cheerful spirit.

The next time we plan a pity party, we should decide to not participate. Throw a thank you party instead. Thank you, Lord for changing our focus and letting us rely on You when our strength is gone.

Gratitude replaces pity every time, and it's a lot more fun. Try it; you'll like it.

Prayer: Lord, help me to have an attitude of gratitude. You are so good to me.

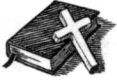

January 12

FAR from God

Do not be quickly provoked in thy spirit, for anger resides in the lap of fools. Ecclesiastes 7:9 NIV

Are you eating everything in sight? Are you restless in your thoughts and your worship? Do you feel empty and worthless? Are you FAR from God?

F – Frustrated
A – Angry
R – Resentful

Compulsive overeating invites other sins. It adds demons to harass your mind and turns you into a fool.

Only God's strength destroys those feelings and compounds worth to your life. Turn your powerlessness to God, and He will release HIS power into your life. First, you must draw NEAR unto God.

N – Newness of mind
E – Energized
A – Amicable
R – Restful

You will marvel at the difference.

Prayer: Lord, help me take time for You today, so that I might feel Your closeness.

January 13

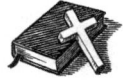

Am I Crazy?

For God hath not given us the spirit of fear; but of power, and of love, and of a sound mind. 2 Timothy 1:7

Have you applied this verse to your life? Is your mind sound? Do you eat things you swore to yourself you wouldn't eat even though you feel terrible afterward? Do you keep eating until you're sick, knowing what's going to happen? Is your life out of control?

The devil seeks to destroy us. Compulsive overeating is one of his prized tools. He brings in his demons of depression, inactivity and worthlessness and has us doing and saying things we would have never believed possible. We might contemplate suicide. We might believe our families are better off without us.

That, my friend, is not a sound mind. You become afraid of yourself with no power to change, but, as the above verse states, "FOR GOD . . . ." Only He has the answer.

Prayer: Today, Lord, give me a sound mind to serve You.

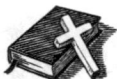

January 14

H.A.L.T.

Come to me, all you who are weary and burdened, and I will give you rest. Take my yoke upon you and learn from me, for I am gentle and humble in heart, and you will find rest for your souls.
Matthew 11:28, 29 NIV

When we follow the Lord, He enriches our lives and leads us to peace of mind and joy of heart. We eat healthy, exercise and worship God with vigor because we're renewed. Then, we flounder again. What could be wrong?

Some of you have heard the expression to HALT and check yourself, but it may bear repeating.

H – Hungry – Have you not eaten enough, or are you letting yourself get too hungry before your next meal? Have you been in the heat or exercised more without food first?

A – Angry – Examine your thoughts. Has someone angered you, but you refused to let it bother you? Did you hide it deep in your mind? It may still be there, causing a desire to overeat.

L – Lonely – Have you spent too much time alone? Does it seem everyone's deserted you? Look around you. Who do you know that might use your help or your company? Let God lead you to the right person.

T – Tired – Have you become too tired, done too much, not gotten enough rest at night? Have you been sick? Have you restored your strength completely before running again?

We must examine our lives. Any and all of these things could hit us, and when it hits compulsive eaters, we want to eat. We may not understand the cause, but we know that's what happens. We should ask God to show us if we need to HALT and take His easier yoke.

Prayer: Open my mind to see the problem, Lord, so I can turn it over to You.

January 15

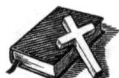

Beauty For the Meek

For the Lord taketh pleasure in his people: he will beautify the meek with salvation. Psalms 149:4

What is the meaning of meek? Webster's says it means submissive. As we submit to God, He dresses us in beauty.

A young woman prayed at the altar last Sunday. I watched her walk down the aisle. I saw the furrows in her brow as she frowned, but after she prayed, her face glowed. Burdens were gone. She walked away a free woman. Though her eyes were tear-stained, she looked beautiful.

When we overeat, we neglect the mirror. Feeling ugly and fat, we turn away from any reminder of our size. We become the picture-taker, so we're not in the photos ourselves. After a time of following a good eating plan, we're not so conscious of the mirror or the camera. The battle is in your mind before it's on the body.

God tells us He "takes pleasure" in us. He loves us as a father loves his children. Through His eyes, we're beautiful. Drawing close through prayer and seeking God's will gives us His viewpoint.

Prayer: Guide my mind to see my beauty through God's eyes.

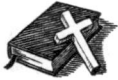

January 16

Who's Your Master, Baby?

Everything is permissible for me—but, not everything is beneficial. Everything is permissible for me—but, I will not be mastered by anything. 1 Corinthians 6:12 NIV

Something or someone masters each of us. We dislike that thought. In verses nine and ten, Paul lists sins that can master us. He includes sexual immorality, idolatry, adultery, homosexuality, prostitution, theft, alcohol, slandering or swindling. All of these are things that hurt our body, our mind, and/or our spirit.

Some people can handle things that aren't sin, but others of us must be watchful. Paul indicated that he could eat meat given to gods. This same meat would condemn other believers. We could use the same excuse for eating a pan of fudge. That would be permissible to us, but not beneficial. The fudge would hurt us since it could overcome our walk with God. God protects us from overeating only while we follow His precepts and commands.

Remember, God gives us rules for our good.

Prayer: Lord, help me remember some foods may be permissible, but let me know if it's not beneficial.

January 17

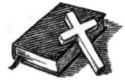

Thank God For the Curse of an Overeating Compulsion?

Always giving thanks to God, the Father, for everything, in the name of our Lord Jesus Christ. Ephesians 5:20 NIV

A friend, Linda, suffered a stroke three years ago. She struggles over simple moves.

"Are you angry with God?" I asked her one day.

Her eyes widened. "Why would I be angry with God when He saved my life and helped me walk and move and sent me a husband who stayed by my side?"

Would I be that gracious? Would you?

Compulsive overeaters tend to blame God. We ask why we were cursed with an inability to control food. We see others that eat candy (like my ex-sister-in-law), or always have dessert (like my mother) and remain slim. Even after receiving an emotional healing, we may fight a compulsion to binge eat because we think we're deprived.

With God's healing, He accelerates our compassion for the lost and addicted. He uses us to assist and pray for others. We travel different roads because we understand the addictive personality. How could we be mad that this curse happened to us when, because of it, God gives blessings?

God desires what's best for His children. We must trust this even when our minds see only negative.

Prayer: Help me trust You and watch for the good.

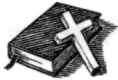

January 18

Taste and Trust

O taste and see that the Lord is good; blessed is the man that trusteth in him. Psalms 34:8

Several Scriptures speak of eating the Word. This one steers us to tasting the Lord. A standard joke, especially among women when we eat too much, is "I'll wear this cheeseburger on my hips tomorrow." Though said in jest, food that we consume becomes part of our bone, our blood, our muscle. Food provides the building blocks of our entire body.

Likewise, what we read, talk about, see on the screen, anything we take into our minds affects our thoughts, our actions, our responses.

What did you taste today?

Where did you place your trust?

The New International Version translates trusting God into taking refuge. That brings a vision of mean people shooting at us. We spot a cave and hide. God is our cave, our refuge from the temptation to overeat. When we can't trust ourselves to do what's right, we can trust God to make it right. Taste (Hide) yourself in Him. The bullets are flying.

Prayer: Today, strengthen my trust and my desire to taste of God's protection.

January 19

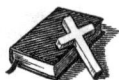

Fear of humiliation

Do not be afraid, you will not suffer shame. Do not fear disgrace, you will not be humiliated. You will forget the shame of your youth and remember no more the reproach of your widowhood. Isaiah 54:4 NIV

Unkind words and prejudice in the work place can bring us humiliation. Have you been passed over for a job because you were fat? Has anyone asked you when your baby was due when you were not pregnant? Has bitter resentment or low self-esteem isolated you from friends?

God gives us the above promise. We can hold up our heads and forget the shame of the past. God's heart breaks because of our pain. He wants to hug us and tell us there is hope, but we won't let Him.

If you're plagued by feelings of disgrace or a desire to hide and eat, call on God. Instead of asking Him to stop the cravings, ask Him to take control. We tire of fighting the battle with little success. The fact is we're powerless. God has all power to "take away the shame of our past and cause us to forget the reproach of our weight."

Prayer: Lord, I come to You today and lay my humiliation and inability at Your feet.

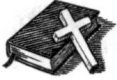

January 20

I Have the Answers to Overcome

May the Lord cut off all flattering lips and every boastful tongue that says, We will triumph with our tongues, we own our lips— who is our master? Psalms 12:3,4 NIV

Most of us begin diets at a young age and then try every new plan that hits the market. We study pamphlets, read books, sit under every type of teaching about weight control. We learn to quote the nutritional value of most foods. Many of us consult psychiatrists or psychologists. Still, our emotional deficiency drives us to overeat.

Our conversation goes:

"I know it all. I can handle it."

"I've lost weight, so I've proven I can do it."

God warns in the Bible that pride is deadly. How many times have we failed because we trusted ourselves? In most nutritional ways of eating, newbies can lose weight rapidly, but those of us who've done it before lag, lose slowly, or not at all. Why? Because we think we know it all.

I am not the master of my fate, nor the captain of my soul. Only God can overcome the beast that food becomes in my life.

Prayer: Lord, though I know a lot, I can't do it. Take over my compulsive eating.

January 21

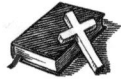

Is God Enough?

Cast your cares on the Lord and he will sustain you, he will never let the righteous fall. Psalms 55:22 NIV

Webster's dictionary gives the meaning of sustenance as food or nourishment. Is God enough nourishment to keep us alive? Not exactly. He made our bodies to require physical food, but only God can provide for the spiritual.

The spiritual and the physical are more closely related than one might think. Without adequate spiritual replenishment, compulsive overeaters eat the wrong things and eat too much, or binge and purge. Anorexics eat too little without God's help.

Clarity comes when we read the definition of sustain—to carry the weight of, or support, to endure and withstand. When we call on the Lord, He sustains (supports, carries) us. Interesting thought.

To a person whose thoughts dwell too much on food, the last phrase in that verse is like the cherry on top of a luscious dessert. God never fails. **He never lets us fall**. Oh, thank you, Jesus.

Prayer: Today, I cast my cares on You, so You can sustain me without failure.

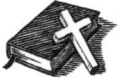

January 22

Hypocrites

Therefore, rid yourselves of all malice, and all deceit, hypocrisy, envy and slander of every kind. 1 Peter 2:1 NIV

Speaking of ourselves as hypocrites is the last thing we want to do. Hypocrites in the church can block seekers from salvation. Until I turned 16, my father remained unsaved because of them. He owned service stations and watched many who attended church cheat and lie in business. He didn't want any part of those hypocrites.

Upon examining our lives, we face guilt. Hypocrisy isn't something way out there. The more healing God brings to our emotions, the more we realize hypocrisy is in us.

Honesty and a genuine desire to serve God may permeate most of our lives. Occasionally, our minds build strongholds that we refuse to give to God. Do you find that after praying in church, you seek solace in food, giving it the place that God should have owned?

The devil fights our minds. It's his favorite and most successful battlefield. The Bible tells us he goes to and fro on the earth seeking to destroy. He knows each of our weaknesses. He knows we won't kill anyone, and we won't commit adultery. Ah, but he also knows if he causes our minds to obsess over a food product, God loses us as His true followers. If we replace God on the throne of our mind, the devil wins. Our Christian walk falters as effectively as if we had lied or cheated.

Prayer: Lord, keep me from being a hypocrite and keep my mind on You.

January 23

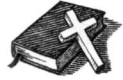

Take these Chains

If the Son therefore shall make you free, ye shall be free indeed.
John 8:36

A chorus we often sing in church goes "my chains are gone, I've been set free." When we lay this compulsive eating disorder into God's hands, that's the way we feel. That's the way it is.

Sin and addiction ties us in knots. Chains bind us, often for years, despite all our intentions to the contrary; chains of self-hate, resentments, inadequacies, and overeating. Our power, our will cannot break them, but Jesus, sweet Jesus, sets us free, really free.

As long as we rely on Him, our minds don't labor over what to do. He chooses our path. We only need to lean on Him. Christ's freedom grows stronger during our difficult periods.

His strength in our weakness—now there's something worth rejoicing about, today.

Prayer: Thank you for true freedom. Help me not to go back to the chains.

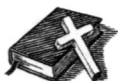

January 24

His Burdens are Light

For my yoke is easy and my burden is light. Matthew 11:30

Jesus' words give hope. When we take over the control of our life, we become weighed down and overwhelmed. Burdens war in our minds. We become exhausted. Verse 28 of that same chapter starts with Jesus calling to all the weary and overburdened. That's us when we control our lives. But, when we lay our heavy load at Jesus' feet, we walk away under His yoke, and His yoke is easy.

Recently, day after day, my mind strained against a heaviness. Troubles wore me down with cares. I was bone tired. When I called on Jesus' name, He didn't fail me. He lifted that load and replaced it with peace. Why do I continue to forget that and allow myself to take over the control of life? I always fail.

Has this happened to you? Ask God for EASE. Remember.

> **E**ase my burden
> **A**dmit my attempted control
> **S**ubmit to His will
> **Y**oke – Mine is harsh, His is light

Prayer: Relieve my heaviness today, Lord. Take over the controls.

January 25

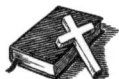

My Strength is Gone

The Lord will judge his people and have compassion on his servants when he sees their strength is gone . . .
Deuteronomy 32:36

An older woman with arthritic hands may have problems opening jars. Still, she works at it. She tugs and twists. She uses a rubber pad to grip the jar or heat it on a burner to loosen the top. That's me. When all else fails, I give it to my husband. He grins and says, "All you had to do was ask." Then he opens the jar.

We're like that with God. We lay awake at night trying to bring a solution for our child, our friend, or us. Trying several things that end in failure, we finally give up and go to God with our problem in our hands. Don't you envision him grinning and saying, "All you had to do was ask." Then He works out the problem.

Too often, we do this with compulsive overeating. We follow one diet after another. We count carbs, and points and calories, then we go on a binge of eating. We hold pain in our hearts.

"Lift our useless attempts and our heartache," we pray.

God says "All you had to do was ask." And, He releases us from the compulsion.

Prayer: Lord, my strength is gone. I need Your compassion and help.

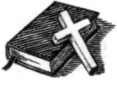

January 26

I Will Wait

I say to myself, 'The Lord is my portion, therefore, I will wait for Him.' Lamentations 3:24 NIV

Waiting is the hardest thing we do. Recently, while heating a leftover dinner in the microwave, I became perturbed that I had to keep putting it back for more seconds. When would it be hot? Laughter broke up my irritation when I thought how I used to heat leftovers on the stove or in a conventional oven. Those methods took three to four times longer to heat, and tasted worse.

We're an instant-type society.

Instant gratification—wanting what we want when we want it—not wanting to wait. That impatience creeps into our relationship with God. If financial problems don't come with an immediate resource, if our kids don't live the way they should, if we follow a diet to the letter and don't drop pounds in three days, we blame God. Why doesn't He answer our prayers?

What does "my portion" in the above verse mean? Webster defines it as one's fate or share. I think of it as hope, our future. God is our fate. He's who we want to shape our life. Therefore, we will wait.

Trust = hope = wait

Prayer: Lord, one of the fruits of the Holy Spirit is patience. You are my fate. Help me to wait.

January 27

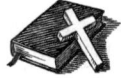

Call Me A Mule

Do not be like the horse or the mule, which have no under-standing, but must be controlled by bit and bridle, or they will not come to you. Psalms 32:9 NIV

Rebellion causes us trouble.

Why am I surprised that my children are rebellious? I've been their example. I have a healthy way of eating planned. When I turn away from it, the Lord has to put a bit in my mouth to bring me back to Him. Being a mule or a jackass isn't a pretty picture, but often I qualify.

Recently, family problems baffled my mind. I prayed and prayed, but things got worse. Anger crept into my thoughts. I quit praying. That lasted three days. I missed my daily spiritual meals.

I was miserable, so I decided to tell God about it. "Lord, I'm mad at you. I need help here, and You're not doing Your part."

God told me, "Well, when you get through having your temper tantrum, you'll be able to see my answers." He was right. My mulish ways blinded me to the truth. God was working. I needed to remove the bit and follow.

The Lord tells us to refrain from acting like a mule or horse. Rebellion creeps into all areas of our walk with God, but most of all in our eating. Observe the mule. Kick bad attitudes.

Prayer: Lead, and I will follow. Feed me, and I will partake.

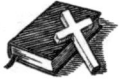

January 28

Resentment Destroys Peace

A sound heart is the life of the flesh; but envy the rottenness of the bones. Proverbs 14:30

In the Big Book of Alcoholics Anonymous as well as Overeaters Anonymous, we read "resentment is the number one offender. From it stems all forms of spiritual disease, for we have been not only mentally and physically ill, we have been spiritually sick."

The two men who started this twelve-step program in the 1930s received their wisdom from the Bible. Note in the verse from Proverbs, envy (resentment or jealousy) rots our bones. Only the Lord can remove these feelings from our minds and restore us to a sound mind and heart, but God will not free us without our consent. We must ask and be genuinely desirous to be free of the envy.

First, we ask God to reveal any bitterness or resentful attitude. Second, we release it to God. In some cases, we must apologize or attempt to reconcile with the person we envied or resented. Sometimes the first person we must forgive is ourselves. When we do our part, God rushes in with sweet peace and acceptance.

Prayer: Lord, show me any resentments and remove them from my mind today.

January 29

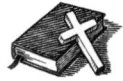

Helping Others Help Us

Who comforteth us in all our tribulation, that we may be able to comfort them which are in any trouble, by the comfort wherewith we ourselves are comforted of God. 2 Corinthians 1:4

The twelfth step in the Alcoholics Anonymous Big Book states "Having had a spiritual awakening as the result of these steps, we tried to carry this message to alcoholics, and to practice these principles in all our affairs."

Alcoholics Anonymous saved our aunt and uncle from a lifetime of alcohol abuse. We watched while their lives were consumed with meetings and service. As the twelfth step says, they couldn't stay sober without trying to help others to stay sober. Bill W and Dr. Bob, who started that organization in the 1930s, soon realized that the only way they could stay away from their own vice was by helping others overcome their addiction.

Christ told of this principle long before Bill W and Dr. Bob learned it. The verse above tells us that when we receive comfort (assistance, inspiration, salvation), we should offer it to others. No one can understand the problem of compulsive overeating like another bound by the problem. We've been there. We know the difficulty.

Notice that this isn't a commandment to tell someone else how to handle their compulsion. What works for me won't work for someone else. Our job to point them to the One who can advise them. Offer Jesus daily to needy souls.

Prayer: Send someone my way today that needs Your comfort.

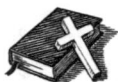

January 30

Having Patience Is the Pits

For ye have need of patience, that, after ye have done the will of God, ye might receive the promise. Hebrews 10:36

God will always bring about His plan and fulfill His promises. God wants us healthy and in tune with Him. Our part is to give the problem to Jesus, ask for His strength, take baby steps toward nutrition. God will do the rest.

Ah, but patience—therein lies the problem. We hate to wait for anything. We are the generation of microwaves, fax machines and high-speed internet. During our journey of weight loss, patience and trust intertwine. If we trust God completely, if we believe we will receive the promise, all we can do is wait.

How long does it take to lose 100 pounds? Many accomplish this in less than a year. I lost ninety-five pounds, but it took me 2 ½ years. Patience grows through the process of trusting God when things look bleak. Have you had a trial in patience lately? Have you faltered and gained? Have you held in your angry words and instead stuffed your mouth with candy? Have you stayed on your eating plan, but not lost any weight?

God is faithful. He keeps His promises. Have you relied on Him?

Prayer: Lord, help me to trust in You today and do my part.

January 31

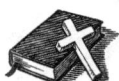

What's Right About Me?

I will praise thee; for I am fearfully and wonderfully made; marvelous are thy works; and that my soul knoweth right well.
Psalms 139:14

Consider listing your talents, your good points, your strengths. This assignment can change your life.

Near the beginning of my weight loss, my mentor asked me to list ten things I liked about myself. This was one of the hardest tasks I'd ever undertaken. Writing things I disliked would've come easily. I was fat, rebellious, stubborn, a control freak . . . I could go on and on.

For an example, here's how my process went:

1. I'm a good mother. No, I yell at my kids too much especially when I'm *drunk* with too many sweets. I marked that out.

2. I'm faithful to my husband. Yes, but . . . my husband suffers from my terrible mood swings. My husband entertains with a fat wife. It was hard. My teacher said start with physical attributes. All mine were bad.

"Well, my eyebrows are dark."

"Think harder," my teacher said.

Finally, I came up with a good list.

Try this today. God's works are marvelous, even our creation. The list will encourage you and lift your self-esteem.

Prayer: Lord, when I get down on myself, remind me of the good things You ascribed to me.

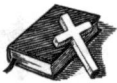

February 1

One Day At a Time

Give us this day our daily bread. Matthew 6:11 The Lord's Prayer

Jesus provided His disciples with an example of how to pray. When we go to that pattern, we learn many lessons. Today, let's look at verse eleven of this prayer. Jesus didn't advise us to pray that God fulfill all our needs forever. His example says to pray for what we need day by day.

A faith walk comes one step at a time. As an only child, I made all the decisions and did the multitude of things needed when my mother died. At the same time, I dealt with my grief as a daughter. While I soaked my husband's shirt with tears for the umpteenth time, I said, "Why can't God heal the wounds once and for all, and then I'd be okay?" But, the pain and indecision came in waves. So does life.

We're a leaky sieve. We can't hold a life's worth of God's provision. We learn and grow a little at a time, like a kinder-gartner who isn't ready for high school graduation.

It does no good to worry about tomorrow's strength or being deprived of our favorite dish at Christmas. We should rely on the Lord today, maybe even one hour at a time.

Prayer: Lord, give me my daily strength and provide the power I lack for now.

February 2

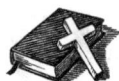

My Tightfisted Control

Whereas ye know not what shall be on the morrow, For what is your life? It is even a vapour that appeareth for a little time and then vanisheth away. For that ye ought to say, If the Lord will, we shall live and do this, or that. James 4:14,15

Let's get this straight. Who's in control of our lives?

Like a director in a play, we position our husbands here, our children and their spouses in a perfect world, and our grandchildren are to play the angel part. When one of them steps out of line, we fume and lay awake nights trying to decide how to make them change. As if we could direct other people's lives, when we can't even control our own.

The more control we try to exert, the worse our drama unfolds.

God is sovereign. When we least suspect, He may allow our Play-Doh figurines to be squashed and our world turned topsy-turvy.

As the verse says, our life is pure steam. Puff, and it's over. If we will release our tight fists, the Lord will take over and guide us. There's such freedom in not being in control anymore.

Prayer: Lord, humble Your servant to submit to Your direction.

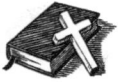

February 3

Fear of Falling

For thou has delivered my soul from death; wilt not thou deliver my feet from falling, that I may walk before God in the light of the living? Psalms 56:13

We pray for our children. God assures us of His answering through His Word and through peace after our prayer.

Recently, I had an unusual assurance from God in the form of a dream. A lady stood at the back of my church handing out peanut butter and jelly sandwiches to everyone who entered. She blessed each one as she handed them a sandwich. Another lady stood at the platform to teach. Her hair burst into fire. She just smiled and continued her talk, so the fire obviously didn't hurt her. God reminded me if He could allow sandwiches to be passed out in church and could set a woman on fire without pain, He could do anything, including save my children.

Fear overwhelms us when we start a weight loss program. We fear we won't lose weight. We fear we'll mess up—again. We even fear we'll lose the weight and then be a different person.

God wants us to believe that if He can deliver our souls from death and save us from hell, He can surely keep us from falling on a weight loss journey. God is a gentleman. He gave us free will, and He will not cross that line. It's up to us to put the control of our eating in His hands.

Prayer: Lord, I believe You can keep me from falling. Help Thou my unbelief.

February 4

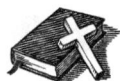

I Don't Have Time to Pray

The Lord will fight for you; you need only be still.
Exodus 14:14 NIV

When our to-do list for the day stretches farther than our hourly allowance, we're tempted to bypass time to visit with God. An extra hour to work could help. Besides, relaxing our minds will be difficult.

What really happens if that's what we do?

We delve immediately into chores. The computer won't work. The phone rings off the wall with petty issues. We can't find our needed workbook. At the end of the day, we're stressed, frustrated, angry and want to eat everything in sight.

When we're busy, more reasons abound for not neglecting our quiet time in the morning. Methods vary for this special time. Here's a suggestion to consider:

1. Focus on Jesus, His faithfulness, His goodness.
2. Praise His name. Thank Him for His blessings.
3. Ask Him for help with your day, for His peace and direction in all that you do.
4. Send up your petitions and intercede for others.
5. In the quiet and peace of that moment, listen for His voice.
6. Close the prayer by asking for His will, His choices to be done that day in your life.

We must not allow the devil to tempt us to give up this time or deceive us into thinking we'll never relax enough to pray. In the garden, God searched for Adam to walk and visit with Him, but Adam got in trouble and hid. God still calls us to spend time with Him.

Prayer: I hear you calling, Lord. Remind me I need to visit with
You before I tackle the world's cares.

35

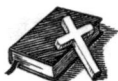

February 5

Me, a Slave?

I put this in human terms: because you are weak in your natural selves, just as you used to offer the parts of your body in slavery to impurity and to ever-increasing wickedness, so now offer them in slavery to righteousness leading in holiness.
Romans 6:19 NIV

In America, we raise independent children. We want them to stand on their own feet. We shudder at the thought of being a slave to anyone or anything. Because of our civil war, black Americans were freed from slavery. Later, we gave women equal rights to vote and hold office.

This independent spirit can backfire. Our stiff-necked thinking refuses to be dependent, even on God. For compulsive overeaters, following our wills can lead to extra pounds and, ultimately, death.

What is God saying through Paul in the above verse? Who was God calling slaves? He didn't mean people owned by another person. Webster's definition of slave: One dominated by other's influence.

Many things dominate our lives—some bad, but many good. If we make a list of possible capturers or things that enslave, it might include: drugs, alcohol, smoking, overeating food or avoidance of food, work, fishing, golf, football, luxury home, automobile, sex, movies, dancing, a person, even church work.

Anything we put on the throne of our hearts in place of God, anything we devote our time and attention to, anything influencing our thoughts and behaviors, to that we become slaves. As the Scripture says, "We are weak."

"If you don't stand for something, you'll fall for anything."
R. O. Thornton

Prayer: Lord, make me Your slave today.

February 6

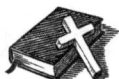

Remember the Past, or Not?

The rabble with them began to crave other food, and again the Israelites started wailing and said, If only we had meat to eat. We remember the fish we ate in Egypt at no cost—also the cucumbers, melons, leeks, onions and garlic. But now we have lost our appetite; we never see anything but this manna.
Numbers 11:4-6 NIV

When we hit a rough spot in life, we sometimes look at how much better the past seemed. Time covers memories of the bloated stomachs, aching heads and numbing depression that we suffered when we binged on sugary, salty, or high-fat foods.

God supplies vegetables and fruits, lean meats, and whole grains. We are not deprived. Still, we forget His provision when we think of past treats, just as the Israelites tired of the manna.

Should we stop to remember the past, or not? Dwelling on the past can have both good and bad consequences.

The reality is that the past wasn't always beautiful. The future with God's direction is peace, love and joy. One day of submitting to a driving compulsion can highlight the difference. One day of overindulgence spurs our thought to the sluggish, hopeless mindset of giving into addiction.

What is *bad* about looking at the past?
- Glamorizing the *good* foods we used to enjoy.
- Dwelling on the tastes and not the effects.

What is *good* about looking at the past?
- Seeing God's grace.
- Receiving feedback on what did and didn't work.
- Inspiration to NEVER GO BACK.

Prayer: Help me use the past and look to You for power, for direction, for answers.

37

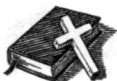

February 7

Honesty

Providing for honest things, not only in the sight of the Lord, but also in the sight of men. 2 Corinthians 8:21

Our older relatives, including my dad, love to quote one-sentence bits of wisdom. One of Dad's favorites was "honesty is the best policy." Freedom from compulsive overeating requires rigorous honesty with ourselves, which is often the hardest task.

The compulsive personality seeks perfection in everything around us. Too easily, we find fault with a husband who's never around, a boss who makes us feel useless, or a friend who doesn't understand. God gives us authority to change only one person. To each of us, He gave a free will, and God will not cross that will.

In the twelve-step program of Overeaters Anonymous, the first step is to admit we are powerless over food. As an independent, strong person, that kind of honesty can nearly break us, but without it we can't heal. Salvation comes with an honest admission that we have sinned with our eating and our attitudes. We stand in need of God's power to cleanse us.

Be honest regarding your compulsions and your need for God.

Serenity Prayer: Lord, grant me the serenity to accept the things I cannot change, the courage to change the things I can, and the wisdom to know the difference.

February 8

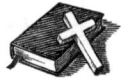

Eat What Is Good

Why spend money on what is not bread, and your labor on what does not satisfy? Listen, listen to me, and eat what is good, and your soul will delight in the riches of fare. Isaiah 55:2 NIV

Americans super-size insatiably. The extra sugar and salt producers add to our foods cause us to crave more and more.

Only we can control what we eat. Yes, I agree, restaurants add extra fats for flavor, processed foods stay good longer, even vegetables get sprayed with pesticides, but we make the ultimate choice. We hold the fork.

The smarter selection is as un-processed as possible. Shop more frequently for produce, perhaps even in the organic section or health food store. Use your own spices to flavor. Salsa adds flavor without fat. Mrs. Dash adds taste without salt. Pass by the lunchmeat and choose chicken or lean beef to cook for your brown-bag lunches. Cook at home more. Make your own low-calorie desserts, or do without. Choose restaurants that offer better low-fat options and post the nutritional values. You DO ultimately control what you eat. They want to please their customers. Let them know what you want.

A sweet roll or donut in the morning increases hunger by mid-morning. A bag of chips for lunch accelerates our desire for a candy bar in the afternoon.

The verse asks, why do you spend money and time getting foods that do not satisfy? When God first created the Garden of Eden, He provided foods to help our bodies operate at peak efficiency. Don't give your body junk and expect the energy, strength and good attitude that you need to serve God. As with computers, it's garbage in, garbage out.

Prayer: Today, help me choose my foods and pastimes wisely so that I'm a better servant for You.

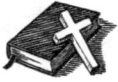

February 9

Watch Out For Yourself

Why do you look at the speck of sawdust in your brother's eye and pay no attention to the plank in your own eye?
Matthew 7:3 NIV

We love comparisons. When we choose to refuse dessert but someone else gets pie, we feel superior. Though we may later commiserate with them, we lift our chins in pride.

Compared to the right people at the right time, we appear holy. Compared to God's righteousness, we're viewed as filthy rags. The verse above was meant to use human reasoning. We must look at ourselves, not someone else—not the overweight, the sinner, the addict—just us.

Our walk with Christ is individual, personal and ours alone.

- Have we given everything to God?
- Our bitterness?
- A son or daughter?
- A condemning mother?
- Unfulfilled dreams?
- A friend's betrayal?
- Envy?
- Our favorite food?

The old song goes "Not my mother, not my brother, but it's me, oh, Lord, standing in the need of prayer."

Prayer: Show me the way set for me.

February 10

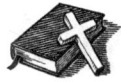

Conceited

And lest I should be exalted above measure through the abundance of the revelations, there was given to me a thorn in the flesh, the messenger of Satan, to buffet me, lest I should be exalted above measure. 1 Corinthians 12:7

Notice that Paul put in, "Don't be exalted above measure," or don't be conceited, two times in one verse. Talk about hitting us over the head.

Helen Keller was quoted as saying "I thank God for my handicaps for, through them, I have found myself, my work, and my God."

The next time we find ourselves thinking "Why did I have to battle with obesity? Why can't I eat like others and not gain weight? Why can't I just quit eating candy or chips or whatever tempts me?" we should bow our heads and say a prayer of thanksgiving for this problem.

Count your blessings. Lest we "exalt ourselves above measure," we were given a propensity to obesity, a compulsion we couldn't control. Thank God that's the biggest problem we face. Only by God's grace does compassion flow from us to others with any type of addiction problem. Only through God.

Prayer: Thank you for giving me the problem of compulsive overeating to hold me back from excessive pride.

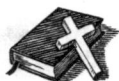

February 11

Are You a Fool?

Do not deceive yourselves. If any one of you thinks he is wise by the standards of this age, he should become a fool so that he may become wise. 1 Corinthians 3:18 NIV

We study diet and nutrition. We follow many good food plans. Still, we fail. We do them in our power, our knowledge. But our way doesn't work. Remember the following truths:

1. Follow God's exact instructions moment by moment.
2. Man's wisdom fails every time.
3. Trusting God for weight loss sounds foolish to the world.
4. We win when we lose ourselves.
5. We succeed when we give up (our will, our choices).
6. Become a fool for God and gain His wisdom and truth.

Prayer: Lord, I give up. I know nothing. Show me the way.

February 12

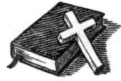

I Am Beautiful

He has made everything beautiful in its time . . .
Ecclesiastes 3:11 NIV

When an extra ninety-five pounds weighed down my body, when more lumps and rolls accented my midsection, I hated mirrors. I wore pants and skirts that wouldn't button, so a big safety pin held them in place under an oversized shirt, but still I was uncomfortable from the tightness. I felt so ugly. I prayed but the heavens seemed as solid as the reflection staring back at me. I hated shopping. I hated dressing up. I hated myself.

But, God says *everything* is beautiful. The words to an old Ray Stevens song uses those same words from Ecclesiastes. "Everything is beautiful. In its own time." No matter how fat or how skinny. Even at our heaviest, God sees us as beautiful since God can see the potential He places within us.

Many things God asks of us can only be done through Him. We must see our beauty while we're still fat, but in our own power, that is impossible. Through Christ, all things are possible—even seeing ourselves as beautiful. I wish for you and for me, today, that we might see ourselves with the eyes of God the Father who formed us, breathed life into us, and presented us to the world as a cherished treasure.

Prayer: Lord, help me see my beauty through You, today.

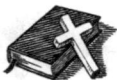

February 13

Don't Let Him Kill Me

The thief comes only to steal and kill and destroy; I have come that they may have life and have it to the full. John 10:10 NIV

The devil is out to kill us. He seeks those who follow Christ. He listens to our conversations and watches for things that tempt us to fall. Life's journey leads over mountains where often we walk close to the precipice. The enemy of our souls searches for opportunity to push us over the edge. The forest of life overshadows us with worry and fear. Valleys sap our determination to look to God.

While fighting a wild fire, firefighters include in their gear a fire shelter for emergencies. They realize that despite all their training and careful planning, situations can fast become more than they can control. In that case, they cover themselves with a flame-retardant protective covering and wait until the fire passes.

God will be our fire shelter if we let Him. When flames of discouragement or temptation threaten to overcome us, God covers and protects. All we need to do is wait for the fire to pass by.

Prayer: Lord, help me to rest under your protective covering and cease trying to fight on my own.

February 14

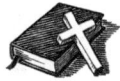

What is Your Spiritual Condition at This Moment?

For this cause we also, since the day we heard it, do not cease to pray for you, and to desire that ye might be filled with the knowledge of his will in all wisdom and spiritual understanding. That ye might walk worthy of the Lord unto all pleasing, being fruitful in every good work, and increasing in the knowledge of God. Colossians 1:9-11

Our ability to stick with the eating and exercising plan we've chosen depends, more than anything, on our spiritual welfare. We don't like to hear that. We resist that idea. We believe we serve God to our utmost. We become angry because God isn't answering our prayers to take off that weight or take away that craving for sweets.

When I reached that point of desperation, I attended a Christian Weight Controllers meeting. I faced my true ugly spiritual status. My self-pitying martyr complex was actually my self-will puffed up and fighting for MY way instead of GOD'S way. When I laid my will at the foot of the cross, Jesus began to work miracles in my physical and mental status. We are three-fold—physical, mental, and spiritual. One affects the other.

Whenever we feel the need to compulsively binge on any food, we need to fall on our knees and pray as Jesus prayed in Gethsemane, "Not my will, but Thine be done." Nothing in ourselves can bring forth the fruit of self-control and pleasing attitude. ONLY GOD.

Prayer: Shine your light on any self-will, self-pitying in me today, else I stumble.

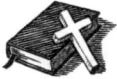

February 15

God's Ways Are Strange

For whoever wants to save his life will lose it, but whoever loses his life for me will save it. Luke 9:24 NIV

I will never understand the ways of God. They aren't man's ways, so they appear strange to us.

If we save, we lose.

If we lose, we save.

If we give up control, we have control.

If we submit our will to God, we're content.

If we give, we gain.

If we hoard, we become empty.

The verse before the one above tells us to "take up our cross daily and follow Jesus." Only through following God's strange rules can we succeed in overcoming any addiction, hurt or hang-up.

Prayer: Lord, help me lose my will, my choices, in Yours.

February 16

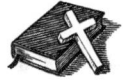

He will Do It

The one who calls you is faithful, and he will do it.
1 Thessalonians 5:24 NIV

When we begin our journey of healing, we should search the Scripture for God's promises to get us through the rough times. Here are my choices:

"God shall supply all your need ..." Philippians 4:19

"... our sufficiency is of God." 2 Corinthians 3:5

"I can do all things through Christ which strengtheneth me." Philippians 4:13

" ... And whatsoever ye shall ask in my name, that will I do ..." John 14:13

God's Word overflows with promises of His love and His provision. He is *El Shaddai* or, as Beth Moore translates it, The Caregiver. Without Him, we're powerless to overcome compulsive overeating.

I can give you several stories of supernatural deliverance. One of my favorite true stories is this: Every morning I picked up a dozen doughnuts on the way to work. No, I didn't have a dozen people there, just me. Within an hour and a half, when another person got to work, I had devoured those donuts. After all, I didn't want any left to prove I bought them for just me.

God delivered me from that habit. I know it was God, because I tried so many times and failed. I've been at the red light, ready to turn into the donut shop, when something captured my attention. The next thing I remember was pulling into my work parking lot right on time with no donuts.

Try it. Even though you plan to overeat, pray and leave it with God to go on about your day.

Prayer: Lord, take over my will, my choices, my compulsion today.

47

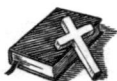

February 17

Thank the Lord, and Get Your Rest

Return unto thy rest, O my soul; for the Lord hath dealt bountifully with thee. Psalms 116:7

The New International Version ends that verse with "the Lord has been good to me." Years after we lose weight, we must remember to thank God for healing us on a continual basis. We must also rest in the belief that He will continue our healing, one day at a time.

Two things overwhelm me with the compulsion to eat too much or eat the wrong foods. The first is becoming too tired or overwhelmed with worry or activities. Set priorities in your life and review them periodically. I don't have the faintest idea why we overload ourselves, but women especially often succumb to that temptation. When we're not resting in the presence of God, the devil gains an inroad. We convince ourselves that candy will energize us to finish our tasks. Instead, sweets depress and slow our effectiveness.

Rest, I say. Rest in the Lord.

The second reason for temptation for me is once more relying on my power, believing I'm doing so good, I don't need God's help anymore. The last time I taught a weight recovery class at church, pride brought me failure. I focused on what I had accomplished instead of what God had done through me.

Thank you, Lord, for helping me. I'm powerless without You.

Prayer: Lord, put up a red flag when I become overextended, or filled with pride.

February 18

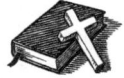

I'm A Lowly, No-good Sinner

I will arise and go to my father and will say unto him. Father, I have sinned against heaven and before thee.
And am no more worthy to be called thy son; make me as one of thy hired servants. Luke 15:18,19

Food immersed me in condemnation. I was fat and unworthy of love. Though I cried out to the Lord for help, I couldn't believe He would heal me because I knew my past actions and vile thoughts. My insecurities and low self-esteem drove me to eat more and more to block out my weaknesses, and then giving in to my compulsion tangled me in a physical and mental addiction.

What a relief to fall on my face and confess to my heavenly father my unworthiness, my inability to overcome the drug that bound my body and mind. The above verse is from Jesus' story of the prodigal son. Later in the chapter (verse 24), the father says, *"For this my son (or daughter) was dead and is alive again, he was lost and is found . . . ."*

We can't trust our history or our ability or even our desires, for all will deceive us at times. Our trust rests only in the Lord's power and love.

Prayer: Today, I worship at the table of my God wherein lies my confidence.

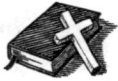

February 19

Where Are My Reins?

Do not be like the horse or the mule which have no under-standing, but must be controlled by bit and bridle or they will not come to you. Psalms 31:9 NIV

Not a pretty picture does God paint in this verse. We don't want to be a horse or mule. When I was a hundred pounds overweight, my doctor called me "a contented cow." Animals have no reasoning capabilities. Humans should make wise choices.

Overeating binges ruin relationships, destroy effectiveness and reduce productivity.

Proper healthy nutrition:

1. Increases your energy level
2. Improves your cognitive skills
3. Heals your body
4. Strengthens your coping skills
5. Buoys your mental attitude

We are better people—Christians, wives or husbands, mothers or dads, daughters or sons, church members, employees and friends—when we practice abstinence in our eating.

Still, we often act like a mule that needs reins to control every action. We're powerless when faced with food.

Prayer: When I'm tempted to overeat, Lord, remind me of the mule who needs reins to come to You.

February 20

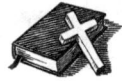

I Don't Like That One

But the fruit of the Spirit is love, joy, peace, longsuffering, gentleness, goodness, faith, meekness, temperance, against such there is no law. Galatians 5:22,23

In a recent Bible study, we named these nine fruits of the Spirit. Everyone forgot temperance. We don't like that one.

Webster gives this definition for temperance: self restraint in conduct, indulgence of the appetites, etc, or moderation.

Nope, I don't like that one.

As I think about the other fruits—love, peace—I realize I can't have God's love or God's peace through my own power. Only the Holy Spirit can reside in us and direct our thoughts and actions and keep them in perfect harmony with God. Why, then, do we think we have to come up with self-restraint all by ourselves? We don't. We can't. Only the Spirit's power working in us can bring forth the fruit of temperance.

Prayer: I abide in Jesus, the vine. He produces the fruit. Thank you, Lord.

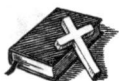

February 21

Keep Climbing Your Ladder

So we say with confidence, the Lord is my helper, I will not be afraid. What can man do to me? Hebrews 13:6 NIV

I am not afraid. Well, maybe a little. When I started this path, I had failed at every weight loss plan known to man or woman. Every time experts discovered a new method, I was on it, hopeful that was my break-through moment.

But on this path, it wasn't some new plan or new food or even a miracle cure but more like a step ladder. Each day, each moment, I scaled the next rung—teetering like a drunk—with God's hand firmly on my back, not allowing me to fall.

Don't wait for that awe moment, and don't wait until you're not afraid. Victory might never come if you wait. Ask for God's help and take a step. God doesn't yank or pull or blind us with a flashing neon sign. He watches. When we move a step, He moves with us.

Have you drug out your ladder? Have you taken the first step? Success comes in steps of faith, not in jumping chasms.

Prayer: I'm taking a step today and trusting You to be beside me because You've never let me down.

February 22

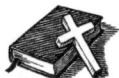

Top Ten Reasons to Let God Control Your Food

And I will make them, and the places round about my hill a blessing, and I will cause the shower to come down in his season; there shall be showers of blessing. Ezekiel 34:26

When we walk in God's will for our eating, showers of blessings fall—some expected, some not.

My personal top ten blessings:

10. I have pride in success or achievement.
9. I look better in my clothes.
8. I have more energy.
7. I eased my leg and back pain.
6. I've learned to like new foods that God has provided.
5. I have lowered my blood pressure.
4. I can board any ride at a fair or Six Flags without worry.
3. I'm able to hike up mountains.
2. I have more self-esteem.

And my all time favorite blessing:

1. I will never again be embarrassed because I can't sit in a tight-fitting restaurant booth.

Can you relate? God specializes in the details and some of the small things are very important to us.

Prayer: Thank you Lord, for the blessings of healthy eating with Your power at the wheel.

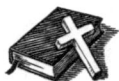

February 23

Who's Your Counselor?

I will instruct you and teach you in the way you should go; I will counsel you and watch over you. Psalms 32:8 NIV

Many compulsive overeaters, including myself, seek counsel and help from psychologists, psychiatrists or licensed social workers. In the throes of depression, we may desire to die.

Through Christian teaching most of my life, God placed within me a fear of going to hell if I committed suicide. This thin thread kept me alive during my roughest period.

Licensed psychologists benefit many. Sometimes, depression requires medicine to control the physical part of the disease. If Christians, they will point us to the source of all truth—Jesus Christ. I didn't go to Christians. One of my counselors undermined my Christian beliefs. I didn't receive help from them.

The emotional imbalance and mood swings common with a true compulsive overeater (not unlike any obsessive-compulsive disorder), though sometimes requiring professional help, must first be given to the one true counselor and teacher. Jesus sent the Holy Spirit to guide us into all truth and knowledge.

Prayer: Lord, teach me, guide me, counsel me.

February 24

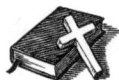

I'm a Natural Rebel

Let us lift up our hearts and hands to God in heaven, and say We have sinned and rebelled . . . Lamentations 3:41-42 NIV

Anytime someone tells me I can't do something, my natural instinct is to do it. Yes, I'm a rebel. During early childhood, I was skinny and sickly, and Mom sought to feed me to health. By pre-teens, my mid-section blossomed, and she began to put me on diets. She was a good mother and only wanted the best. We had plenty to eat, and I enjoyed it all. Dieting became a way of life for me after age fourteen.

When I was told to not eat candy, I kept a stash hidden. When my diet said no donuts, I wolfed them down while driving. Has that happened in your life?

We fail to recognize that our rebellion also extends toward God. God tells us to take all things in moderation. God tells us our bodies are temples. When we abuse our temples, or try to kill ourselves with food, we rebel against God. We need to ask forgiveness and rely on God's guidance in everything we do. In reading the Bible, we learn God focuses on the details in His tabernacle and in nature. If He knows the hair on our heads, He cares what we put in our body for fuel.

Prayer: Lord, within myself, I'm a sinner and a rebel. Forgive me.

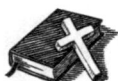

February 25

Are You Ignoring Your Own Truth?

And ye shall know the truth, and the truth shall make you free.
John 8:32

Ask us which is lowest in fat—a cinnamon-raisin bagel or an individual bag of pretzels—and we can give the answer. Ask us for a list of great low-fat snacks, and we'll give suggestions. We know that truth. We know if we don't keep exercising, we'll gain weight again.

Some truth, however, we ignore.

When we want to reset a computer, we turn it off and back on again. Everything reverts to its original settings. Our mind works the same way. We find it impossible to keep on our food plan when our spiritual condition deteriorates. Closeness to God reveals our dependencies and self-defeating habits. Without His light shining on those things, we revert to our years of programming wrong information. "You're worthless. I can't get my mind off food. I deserve a pick-me-up."

We can't afford to bypass our quiet time with our Savior. When we enter His gates of praise and His tabernacle of thanksgiving, He shines His truth on incorrect thinking. We eat what we should. Our day is productive, our mind, content. His truth "sets us free."

Prayer: Today, help me walk in Your truth.

February 26

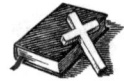

Rebellion in My Mind

Jesus replied; Love the Lord your God with all your heart and with all your soul and with all your mind. Matthew 22:37 NIV

We Christian compulsive overeaters are a stiff-necked bunch, not unlike the Israelites, but God determined to use them anyway and work miracles for them. He made a covenant with the Israelites to do wonderful things in them that other nations could see and give glory to God. No power but God's power can break the bonds of stubborn rebellion.

Jesus gave His number one commandment in the verse above.

We get down the heart, the soul, even the strength. We follow Christ with everything in us, but with our minds, we rebel.

Our minds take in our:

- Reason
- Logic
- Desire
- Imagination
- Memory
- Will

Memory replays old tapes. Our strong wills fight against what God wants. Our reason justifies our desires. Small things grow into a mountain of unbelief and strangle God's will in our lives.

Prayer: Lord, today I seek to love You with all my mind.

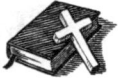

February 27

Jesus Helps Me Because of Himself.

Not by works of righteousness which we have done, but according to his mercy he saved us, by the washing of regeneration, and renewing of the Holy Ghost. Titus 3:5

Failure is my middle name. Like Paul in the Bible, what I want to do, I don't do, and what I don't want to do, that's what I do. In years past, I beat up myself with each fall, but that's not what God wants. Neither does He expect a perfect life. Our own perfectionism buries us in a hole.

God's will is that we realize our humanity, and thereby rest in His arms. God created us. He knows we are dirt. But, He loves us more than we love our wayward children. He asks only that we put our failures and shortcomings into His hands. Jesus lives to intercede for us. When God the Father looks at us, He sees the perfection of His Son. The Holy Spirit supplies strength for us to stay in tune with God because of the goodness of Jesus.

Good thing for us. We don't have to act perfect anymore. We ask Jesus to take over for us. We can't do it alone. What a relief. We can lay down the load we've carried for years. Jesus will pick it up and carry it for us. I'm not perfect. Now, I don't have to act as if I were.

God, You are my sufficiency, my security, my everything.

Prayer: Lord, take over where I falter.

February 28

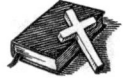

Get Your Sleep and Rely on God

In vain you rise early and stay up late, toiling for food to eat—for he grants sleep to those he loves. Psalms 127:2 NIV

To the person not plagued with compulsive overeating, rising early or staying up late to eat might sound ridiculous, but it happens. Food can become so important to us, so as to even replace rest. After gorging before bedtime, we fall into a fitful slumber only to rise in the morning feeling as if a Mack truck ran over our body, yet our minds yearn for more food to bring rest and give peace.

I know food isn't considered addictive, but from experience, I can tell you it is. My mind and body craved rest from the constant turmoil. I had no peace. I couldn't sleep well at night. I began days feeling sluggish, sleepy and sedated.

If only we gave that much time for communion with the Heavenly Father, we could be a powerhouse for God.

Our bodies need from seven to eight hours of good REM sleep to renovate and revitalize. Are you giving time for healthy fellowship with God, good rest at night and nutritional eating by day?

Prayer: Lord, let Your rest empower me so I can refrain from my compulsion.

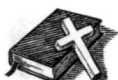

March 1

I Need Peace

Thou wilt keep him in perfect peace, whose mind is stayed on thee: because he trusteth in thee. Isaiah 26:3

Alcoholics Anonymous and all the twelve-step programs say the Serenity Prayer. "Lord, grant me the serenity to accept the things I cannot change, the courage to change the things I can, and the wisdom to know the difference."

God's healing brought me to a place where I believe serenity (peace) is priceless, worth far more than extra food.

Lack of peace negates our Christian witness. Without energy, we lack desire for career accomplishment or an active faith. Our children suffer a sharp tongue simply because we want to be left alone to eat. Our anger assaults our mates though it's meant for us. Without serenity, we become couch potatoes fumbling for mere existence until we can get our next food fix. We are perfectionists that never attain improvement—all because of an overeating compulsion.

True inner peace comes only from the Lord. We can't manufacture it, we can't read our way into it, or act ourselves into calming internal disaster. Serenity is God's gift for us stepping out in faith. We must lean heavily on Him before our next ugly thought, compulsive twinge, or next breath.

Prayer: I trust in You, Lord, for serenity.

March 2

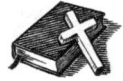

Is My Pride Showing?

When pride comes, then comes disgrace, but with humility comes wisdom. Proverbs 11:2 NIV

God loves a humble and contrite spirit. The biggest problem with perfectionism is we lose that humble attitude. No one does a job to suit us. No one gives the attention we crave. Resentment sprouts its tentacles like an octopus with eight arms. And resentment is a killer for a compulsive person. We stuff a lot of food into our mouths to destroy it. We lash out in anger to hide it. But, still, those multiple arms of resentment suffocate us, wound us, and ultimately ruin our lives.

A simple example would be at the time of my youngest daughter's graduation from high school. Our church gave a reception for the graduates. The organizer gave us parents no instruction of what we might do except the time and place for the party. However, two parents set up bulletin boards highlighting their baby's activities and accomplishments. That was the focus of attention. People passed by my angel's table and book to sign and headed to the *flashy* displays of tribute. (Notice my resentment coming out as I tell the story.) After the reception, I went home, fell on my bed and cried all night. My husband couldn't console me. My daughter thought she'd done something wrong. What should have been a happy time for all evolved into a family nightmare. All because of my resentment.

We can never allow resentment to grow in our minds because the only remedy is food binging.

God's cure:

An attitude of gratitude—otherwise known as "count your blessings."

Prayer: Remove every new sprout of resentment from my mind.

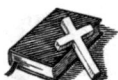

March 3

Moderation? What's that?

Not that I speak in respect of want, for I have learned in whatso-ever state I am, therewith to be content. Philippians 4-11

We hate moderation, and contentment is hard to develop. Our lives focus on too much food, too much work, too much perfectionism, telling the whole story from beginning to end and being all things to all people. Yep, no moderation in our vocabulary.

Where does moderation originate?

A baby drinks as long as we hold the bottle. A child will play until they fall asleep. This moderation thing doesn't come through birth.

Look at the fruits of the spirit. One of them is temperance or self control, others are peace and joy. I believe moderation in all things, as the Bible teaches, comes from the Spirit. Just like faith. Without faith, we can't please God, yet we can't create faith. God gives it to us. Neither can we bring forth moderation.

Compulsive people are the most discontented. Nothing is good enough, especially our own lives. A wheel of disquiet turns in our heads at all times. We replay every bad act, word, or thought over and over like a scratched DVD. The nightmare continues 24/7. Take heart. We are incapable of bringing about calm. Like salvation, that's God's gift, if we will accept it.

Until, God . . . God healed me. God taught me moderation. God produced contentment in my life. Thank you, Jesus. He'll do the same for anyone that's willing.

Prayer: Lord, thank you for contentment right now and continue to show it forth in my life today as I yield to Your will.

March 4

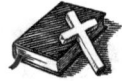

God Doesn't Fail

Because of the Lord's great love, we are not consumed, for his compassions never fail. They are new every morning; great is your faithfulness. Lamentations 3:22,23 NIV

Inconsistency marked my life. For a week, a month, maybe even six months, I would maintain white-knuckled devotion to a diet plan. I counted and measured every bite. Nothing went between my lips that wasn't on my list. Then, it happened. Because of a certain circumstance, I'd eat something wrong. Discouragement brought me to my knees. My thoughts went:

- I messed up.
- What does it matter?
- I can't take this anymore.
- I've already blown it, so I might as well eat something I really want.

After gorging myself for a while, disgust caused me to search for a new plan. Sound familiar?

At this point, every diet seems to fail. Counselors anger us. Even loved ones exacerbate the problem.

God showers us with new compassion every day. He never fails, and He's always there. He's the God of spring after winter, of newborn babies in the face of death, of new years and new songs. He's all we need, fresh every morning.

Prayer: Today, I look to You, the author of something new.

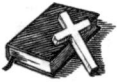

March 5

I'm So Tired

Let us not become weary in doing good, for at the proper time, we will reap a harvest if we do not give up. Galatians 6:10 NIV

Fatigue clamps a tight grip after years of fighting weight. Control slips and ends in disaster. Family members wreak havoc with our emotions. Friends let us down. We take it upon ourselves to make everyone act right but, even as we direct our play, the actors won't keep their rightful places.

Does this despair sound familiar? Compulsive people *need* to heal every illness and restore every relationship. Yet, the more we work at making everything right, the more we fail. No wonder we're exhausted. We're trying to be God, but only He can fulfill that role.

My control = disaster

God's control = freedom

Don't give up, give in! Give in to God. He provides the harvest of sanity, freedom and hope.

Prayer: When I'm tired, take over for me, Lord.

March 6

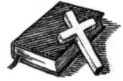

Help Me, Help Me

I am holding you by your right hand—I, the Lord your God—and I say to you, Don't be afraid: I am here to help you.
Isaiah 41:13 Life Recovery Bible

A decision needed to be made that would affect my life for years to come, yet fear froze my forward progress. God gave me the above verse, and some simple instructions:

1. List the pros and cons of your decision.
2. Surrender to God all fear.
3. Follow God's lead without thinking of consequences. Let God handle results.
4. Slow down; breathe easy; enjoy life's little moments of pleasure.
5. Concentrate on the valuable people in your life.
6. Take the first step.

In my case, at that time, the decision was whether to quit my job or not. The first step was to give my boss notice. By taking the first five steps, I was ready for #6.

By following God's instruction, this process didn't throw me into an orgy of overeating, which had been the case during past changes. Thank you, Lord.

Prayer: Lord, lead and help me follow today in whatever might come my way.

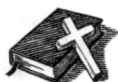

March 7

Like a Child

Whomsoever therefore shall humble himself as this little child, the same is greatest in the kingdom of heaven. Matthew 18:4

One of our daughters couldn't swim. Her sisters, both older and younger, could, but, for months, fear disabled our middle child. Despite this, when her father held out his arms while in the water, she would jump. Though the water scared her, she trusted her dad. Our youngest grandson was also one who stayed on the steps, refusing to venture out unless his dad held him.

To me, that's a visualization of complete trust in Jesus. We stand on the deck, fear immobilizing us, but if we spot Jesus with open arms toward us, we jump.

When a train goes through a tunnel and it gets dark, you don't throw away the ticket and jump off the train. You sit still and trust the engineer. – Corrie ten Boom

Trust a dependable daddy like a child. Though the water is frightening, and the dark is scary, trust Father God.

Prayer: Lead today and I will follow. Beckon today and I will jump.

March 8

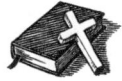

I'm Sowing Seeds and
Preparing for Victory.

Those who sow in tears will reap with songs of joy. He who goes out weeping carrying seed to sow, will return with songs of joy, carrying sheaves with him. Psalms 126:5,6 NIV

Our steps seem small, our successes insignificant. For two days, we eat three healthy, balanced meals with no in-between snacks, but on day three, we add a high-fat meal. What is it we think about the most? That one high-fat meal. For six days, we stay with twelve hundred calories a day then, on the seventh day, we eat a small piece of pie. That pie, in our minds, crowds out all the good.

Don't discount a small seed you plant. Rejoice over leaving a store without candy. Give thanks for God's help in passing McDonald's without a loop through the drive-through. For every party we follow our plan and for every alone-time we focus on something besides food, give God thanks.

I shed many tears over what I thought failure.

God saw the seed I sowed and granted me favor.

Take the steps.

Sow the seed.

Rely on Jesus.

God is responsible for the harvest.

God gives the songs of joy.

Prayer: Lord, gather my seeds today and weave them into a song of joy for tomorrow.

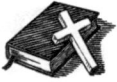

March 9

By Your Spirit

Not by might, not by power, but by My Spirit, says the Lord Almighty. Zechariah 4:6b

Afraid that we'll fail, we shuffle through our day. We swallow huge chunks of vegetables or low-fat foods, trying to fill our stomachs with volume. Knowing we can't choose wisely, we cancel party plans. Our weaknesses shut us inside, doomed to never eat at another restaurant.

Why?

We don't possess the power to withstand temptation anyway. Our might will weaken even if all that's available is frozen waffles or stale cookies.

Victory only comes through God's Spirit, whose guidance and wisdom provide an avenue of success regardless of where we are or what food is there. Rely on Him. Submit your powerlessness.

Prayer: Through Your Spirit, I tread temptation wherever I find it.

March 10

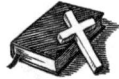

Take Inventory

On October 10 the people returned for another observance; this time they fasted and clothed themselves with sackcloth and sprinkled dirt in their hair. And the Israelis separated themselves from all foreigners. The laws of God were read aloud to them for two or three hours, and for several more hours they took turns confessing their own sins and those of their ancestors. And everyone worshipped the Lord their God.
Nehemiah 9:1-3 Life Recovery Bible

Christian meetings or classes for weight recovery or eating disorders are good tools for compulsive overeaters. Guilt eats at our minds because we eat food according to whim and not in obedience to Christ. As with any other sin, personal confession comes prior to worship. When we meet with Christian compulsive overeaters, we can be honest about what we eat and how much we eat, to God and to other people. Standing in humility and submission frees us for real praise and thanksgiving.

Seek such meetings, if not at your church, perhaps at a twelve-step meeting, or begin your own. Several Christian programs offer such time together to support and encourage others with similar problems. Even Overeaters Anonymous has some totally Christian chapters.

When we go, we should prepare, as the Israelites did in the verse above, to hear from God. Read His Word. Confess compulsions. Praise Him for what He's doing in our lives.

Prayer: Lord, direct me to the meeting You have prepared for me.

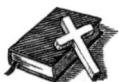

March 11

When Is My Body Safe?

These bodies of ours are constantly facing death just as Jesus did; so it is clear to all that it is only the living Christ within who keeps us safe. 2 Corinthians 4:1 Life Recovery Bible

Our attitude increases our bodies' immunity, improves our circulatory system and lessens our risk of accident. Emotional health and physical health are closely related. In 2 Corinthians, Paul acknowledged the only way to keep our bodies safe from illness and injury comes from Christ. Our praise must float to God from the inside.

Inside our thoughts, we heap praise on God.

Inside our bodies, we serve God in real time.

Inside our hearts, we love with God's insight.

Disease and infirmity lessens our witness. No, we cannot ward off every threat to our health. God allows some things so that we might understand and use the experiences to bring glory to God, or to teach us a lesson. Though God might allow a chronic illness, His will doesn't include continual moaning and complaining.

The more we praise God and let Him control our attitudes, the healthier our bodies become.

Prayer: Lord, I praise Thee from the inside.

March 12

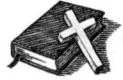

Are you growing?

Forgetting what is behind and straining toward what is ahead, I press on toward the goal to win the prize for which God has called me heavenward in Christ Jesus. Philippians 3:14

God's ideal for us is a perfect Christian walk with no sin, no impure thoughts, witnessing and being always sensitive to God's will in our lives, AND no compulsive overeating.

Perfection is the goal, but we will never reach it. Should we give up because we're not the ideal? No, of course not.

An oak tree strives for the ideal of being tall with many branches giving shade. When we plant an oak in our yard, the height might well be three foot or less. It may have two scrawny branches. Do we cast it aside because it's not perfect? Of course not. We water it, we nourish it, we pray for sunshine and rain at proper times. The oak starts growing. Though slower than many other trees planted at the same time, an oak grows in strength. Life flows through the trunk and branches of an oak at a different pace than through a willow. Yet, we plant and nourish both toward the ideal they can reach.

New Christians are tiny saplings. As more mature Christians, we should help them along, and yet, we also should be growing. If an oak ceases to grow, it ceases to live. Our Christian walk resembles the oak tree. We must stay attached to Christ and continue to grow. Even the mighty full of emotional health must continue to learn and improve.

Are you growing? In your walk with Christ and in overcoming your food addiction? Don't give up.

Poke your head toward the sky and keep striving, regardless that you will never attain perfection until God takes you home. How close can you come?

Prayer: Today, help me stay in You and grow.

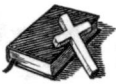

March 13

Don't Think About It

So do not worry, saying 'What shall we eat? Or What shall we drink? or What shall we wear?'But seek ye first his kingdom and his righteousness, and all these things will be given to you as well. Matthew 6:31, 33 NIV

A compulsive overeater spends much time dwelling on what to eat. When we leave for a meeting or visit, we worry that we'll get hungry before we return. For those who have suffered the affects of low blood sugar, that fear is real. When we wait too long to eat, we become dizzy, faint, have throbbing headaches and churning stomachs. Often, we use that possibility as an excuse to mold our lives around our meals.

If we are new to nutrition, we study. We read books, go to classes, or online sites. We might consult a nutritionist. These are good options. We should check out healthy plans like the American Diabetic exchange diet, Weight Watchers, or Bob Greene's The Best Life.

A good food plan includes God's provision without many of man's additions. The Lord's offerings give variety and good taste.

In truth, many of us have studied and dieted for many years. We know what we should eat. When we journey with Christ to healthy weight and emotional health, we should change how often our thoughts remain on food. God says to rest in Him for all things, to seek first His kingdom. He directs our eating into what's best for us, if we lay aside our worry.

Many of us opt for three healthy meals and one light snack. Others need five or six smaller meals strewn throughout the day. Ask God for wisdom. He will direct you. He will provide for you. Seek Him.

Prayer: Today, I seek Your kingdom. Show me what to eat.

March 14

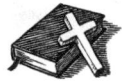

Are You Far from God?

Be careful for nothing; but in every thing by prayer and supplication with thanksgiving, let your requests be made known unto God. Philippians 4:6

Frustration is a tool from the devil used against compulsive overeaters.

✝

Be ye angry, and sin not; let not the sun go down upon your wrath. Neither give place to the devil. Ephesians 4:26,27

Anger needs to be replaced with God's healing, or the devil gains a foothold into the mind of a compulsive overeater.

✝

Remember ye not the former things; neither consider the things of old. Behold, I will do a new thing; now it shall spring forth; shall ye not know if I will even make a way in the wilderness, and rivers in the desert. Isaiah 43: 18,19

Resentment kills the soul of a compulsive overeater.

F – Frustration
A – Anger
R – Resentment

These three sins keep you FAR from God and thereby, keep you bingeing and out of control.

Prayer: Keep me close to You today.

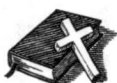

March 15

Deliver Us from Death

Who delivered us from so great a death, and doth deliver; in whom we trust that he will yet deliver us. 2 Corinthians 1:10

We follow a path of death and disease. We mistreat our bodies. The medical field views obesity as a major complication to every illness and surgery. We kill ourselves one bite at time. Though we understand that fact, we pick up the next bite and devour it.

We need a deliverer because our efforts lack power. After years, since God healed me emotionally, I still require protection from my compulsion. Escape comes through God's strength, never through our own because we have none.

Whenever I call on you,
You delivered me nineteen years ago.
You deliver me today.
You will deliver me in the future.
Without God, I am a failure, without strength, without power, without hope.

Prayer: Lord, deliver me now.

March 16

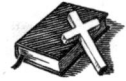

Okay, I'm learning

And patience develops strength of character in us and helps us trust God more each time we use it until finally, our hope and faith are strong and steady. Romans 5:4 Life Recovery Bible

Every time I say "no," it's easier the next time.

Every time I walk out of a store with no extra treats, I win.

Every day I exercise, I up my chances of keeping on with the activity on the next day.

Most of us refuse to pray for patience because we know what lies ahead if God answers—trials. To an individual who battles lack of control where food is concerned, a trial leads to a binge. If we trust in God and take steps as He leads our food intake, we grow in patience, which the Bible tells us develops strength of character.

Every time we hold God's hands and use His strength to take over situations that disturb us and every time He keeps us from overeating, we grow in faith, strength and hope. Yes, each step, no matter how small, counts. Take that first step, then try for another. They add up to freedom.

Prayer: I don't like patience, but I need it. Help me, Lord.

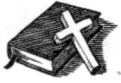

March 17

Liar, Liar, Pants on Fire

Their tongue is a deadly arrow, it speaks with deceit . . .
Jeremiah 9:8a NIV

The Big Book of Alcoholics Anonymous states, "Rarely have we seen a person fail who has thoroughly followed our path . . . They are naturally incapable of grasping and developing a manner of living which demands rigorous honesty."

Because of Adam and Eve, we are born with a sinful nature. Show me a child accused of making a mess that doesn't try to blame his brother or give an excuse for himself. Yes, lying comes with ease. Some people are never able to turn over their lying tongues to God. Yet, without honesty, following Christ is impossible in anything.

The first step to healing from overeating is admitting we can't do it by ourselves. We must give up to God. We might be strong and capable of handling much on our own, but food stumps us. With food, we are powerless.

After this first step, every other step can only be taken with complete lack of deceit to ourselves or others. Every time we battle food, we must shine God's light on our thoughts and actions. We must be totally honest. Has resentment crept into our minds? Are we angry at our brother or sister?

God knows our tongue is a deadly, lying arrow. We must let Him control it.

Prayer: Lord, take over my tongue. Let only honesty reign.

March 18

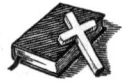

I'm In a Bad Situation

And she called the name of the Lord that spoke unto her, Thou God seest me; for she said. Have I also here looked after him that seeth me. Genesis 16:13

Like Hagar in the story told in Genesis, we might find ourselves in a bad situation, perhaps because of our own choices, or those thrust upon us, as in Hagar's case. Difficulties do not give us the right to go against God's will. As with Hagar, God sees you, and He stands willing to help you.

If we find ourselves in a bad place, we should prove gainsayers wrong, prove by our actions that we can overcome. God watches over us. He provides the escape. A bad situation isn't an excuse for compulsive overeating or another transgression against God's leading.

In Hagar's case, God gave her a command to go back into the fight, relying on Him to get her through it. Eating is something we can't stay away from. We must eat. We must live through the daily struggles. The difference comes from reliance on God.

Prayer: Lord, hold me up even in bad situations.

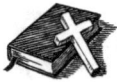

March 19

Wretchedly Wrong

O wretched man that I am, who shall deliver me from the body of this death. Romans 7:24

We put Paul on a pedestal and think of him above temptation. When he lived in the flesh, Paul called himself wretched. We're all human. We all face similar trials and temptations. Whenever we dwell on the carnal and what we want, we are wretched and wrong.

In recent years, we've seen mighty men of God fall from grace. If ever there was a time to remind us of fleshly fame, it would be now. No one is exempt. Why would we expect to be?

Here's an excerpt from my journal:

"I did not realize I was angry. My body translates those feelings into hunger. Those people did nothing wrong. It's me. I'm mad because I didn't stand up for myself. I said 'yes' again when I should've said 'no.' I ate all the candy, now I've started on the cookies and I don't even like them. I'm a mess."

Paul is wretched.

I'm a mess.

My husband worked in retail stores for years. When he took inventory, he might notice an overabundance of men's shirts. He'd overbought. He was forced to admit his mistake by putting them on the clearance table.

What should we face and admit today?

Prayer: Help me to admit my wretchedly wrong behavior.
Clean out the bad stuff and bring in the new.

March 20

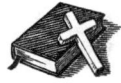

Rumble Strips

Jesus saith unto him, I am the way, the truth and the life, no man cometh unto the Father, but by me. John 14:6

Texas lines its highways with rumble strips to wake sleepy drivers and keep them on the road. Jesus is our highway. For those with a problem of compulsive overeating, He gives warning signs or rumble strips:

1. Trigger foods. We all have foods that we can't tolerate. One bite and we want more. Don't start with these.
2. If cravings or constant desires to overeat nag at you, stop, pray and ask for God's insight into what is bothering you. Many times, we don't know.
3. Never let a day go by without asking for the Lord's help and listening for His guidance.
4. Read God's Word, listen for His instructions, especially during a time of testing.
5. Ask others to help you pray when you're feeling especially out of control or weakened.
6. Be prepared always with good foods you can eat and would enjoy.
7. Do some activity every day unless sickness makes it impossible.

Following these rumble strips keeps sleepy sinners from succulent delights that stagnate success.

Prayer: Lord, keep me aware of the rumble strips you've supplied to keep me on Your road to health.

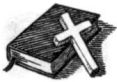

March 21

God lives here?

What? Know ye not that your body is the temple of the Holy Ghost which is in you, which ye have of God, and ye are not your own? 1 Corinthians 6:19

We Christians talk about this body being only a shell. Thereby, we diminish it in importance. When we think of our bodies as a temple for the Holy Ghost, then we look at the oversized, flabby dwelling we supply for Him, and we stand convicted and ashamed.

Tied to a low self-esteem, we use this conviction like guilt and eat more because we feel unworthy. Guilt condemns, but conviction intends to guide us to improvement.

Conviction comes as a gift of God. As weak and faulty humans, our temples are cleaned out by the Holy Spirit when we ask, not unlike Christ cleaned out the money changers from His Jerusalem temple.

Yes, the Holy Spirit lives in us, but it's up to each of us to decide whether we grip the steering wheel of our lives or turn it over to the one inside who is greater.

Prayer: Take over the steering wheel of my body today.

March 22

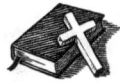

I'm spirit, soul and body.

And the very God of peace sanctify you wholly, and I pray God your whole spirit; and soul; and body be preserved blameless unto the coming of our Lord Jesus Christ. 1 Thessalonians 5:23

The verse above indicates that God desires control of us. He created us in His image as a spirit, soul and body—three parts of a whole—a trinity like God. No one part of us is more important to God's service than the other, just as God, the Father, is no more important than His son, Jesus, or the Holy Ghost.

Take care of the soul by turning it over to God for safe-keeping.

Take care of the spirit (mind) by putting into it wholesome thoughts and deeds in preparation for battle.

Take care of the body by feeding it healthy food and exercising it for strength and endurance.

God puts the whole man into our hands as caretakers for His temple. He desires us to keep it safe for His return. He cares for us. He desires our voluntary worship. He longs to see us realize we can't fulfill all we need to do in this life without His help. One or more of our parts will fail. Have you given to Him your soul, spirit and body?

Prayer: Lord, take all of me.

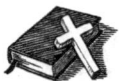

March 23

Crucifixion Comes Before Resurrection

And he saith unto them, Be not affrighted, Ye seek Jesus of Nazareth, which was crucified, he is risen; he is not here; behold the place where they laid him. Mark 16:6

A friend circulated a new Facebook blurb that said, "God is there during your testing time. Remember the teacher remains quiet during a test." I liked that and shared it with my friends. A test during weight recovery may mean a set-back, a temptation or a complete failure for days or weeks.

At this time of year, most Christians reread the Easter story and often hear it taught in church. We see our trials with weight and control through the lens of this holiday. When we step on the scale and realize a significant loss, we rejoice. Our clothes loosen, our energy rebounds and our confidence soars. Reaching goal weight is a time of joyful success.

However, we hate the weeks when we can't lose weight but still feel hungry. We fall on our faces, and think victory will never be ours. God reminds us that even His resurrection could never have happened until He endured the bitter night of arrest, mock trial, the beatings and humiliation. After He walked the road to Golgotha and enemies hung Him to the cross, victory lay ahead.

Remember, until we face our own crosses, we can never have triumph. Even Jesus had to go through the crucifixion before He received His resurrection.

Prayer: Remind me of Your presence during my tests and trials.

March 24

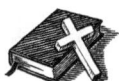

Prayer and Meditation

My heart says of you, 'Seek his face.' Your face, Lord, I will seek.
Psalms 27:8 NIV

Our independence from food addiction comes in direct relation to our dependence on the Lord. That takes daily communication.

Here are the steps I recommend each day:

1. Choose one book in the Bible and read a chapter.
2. Write a letter to the Lord in a journal giving your daily activities, emotions, and problems for the day before. In this way, you release it all to Him.
3. Read a daily devotion such as this or Food for Thought that is based on your own emotional struggles.
4. Concentrate on God—His goodness, faithfulness and strength.
5. Count your blessings. Voice your gratitude to God.
6. Make your petitions for others as well as for yourself.
7. Sit and listen for God's voice to you.

Daily prayer and meditation will hold you safe and steady even when life is traumatic and trying.

Prayer: Lord, I look forward to our daily visits. Help me not forget.

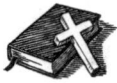

March 25

I Don't Believe I Can

My son, forget not my law, but let thine heart keep my commandments. For length of days, and long life and peace shall they add to thee. Proverbs 3:2

God's word says following his commandments will add peace to our lives. Following them in outward show is not enough. We must agree with our heart. My story may align with overeaters everywhere.

After years of trying to lose weight, my confidence had evaporated. I called out to God but only trusted in my own abilities. Hadn't I been there when I'd lost thirty pounds with a weight support club, only to put it back on plus a little? I'd whittled off forty pounds with shots and pills from a doctor's office to find myself in deep depression and succumbing to the same behaviors that put the weight on in the first place. Then came a new plan. I did so well that I purchased the franchise and operated the business of daily counseling along with a strict diet imposed. The stress of keeping my weight off in public drove me underground to eat huge amounts until I'd gained it all back and had to give up my business.

I knew I failed. I couldn't lose weight. Even if I lost, I couldn't maintain the reduction. How could I ever believe again?

But, what about God?

God promises His peace. He is our confidence. Our success is built on Him. We still can't do it. But, God is faithful. He promises to give peace and a long productive life to all who follow His commandments with their hearts. Ask Jesus what He'd have you eat today.

Prayer: Lord, guide me. You are my confidence.

March 26

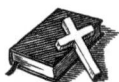

Nope, I Can't Do It

I have been crucified with Christ and I myself no longer live, but Christ lives in me. Galatians 2: 20 Life Recovery Bible

The chapter above goes on to explain that if man could follow the law to salvation, Christ wouldn't have had to die. But, we can't. We're no good at following rules and regulations. Our white-knuckled determination falters when we need it most.

God created us and knew our weaknesses. He loved us enough to send His son to die for us. Then, Jesus sent the Holy Spirit back to earth to reside in Christ's followers, thereby living through us as we submit to Him.

We mere humans stumble over this. We make it hard. We ask the Lord to help us then we grunt and groan, trying to do it ourselves. Excuse my country, but "Ain't gonna happen." Even though we give our hearts to Christ, we still can't lose weight or overcome the addiction to food by ourselves. Only submission, giving up our strong self will, can offer victory.

Prayer: Thank you, Lord, for dying for me. Help me submit today.

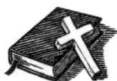

March 27

I Need Something to Hold Onto

O turn unto me, and have mercy upon me; give thy strength unto thy servant, and save the son of thine handmaid. Show me a token for good; that they which hate me may see it, and be ashamed: because thou, Lord, hast helped me, and comforted me.
Psalms 86:16-17

We walk in faith, but we're visual people. We need something to hold in our hands—a token, God calls it, to prove He helps. Two things served that purpose for me.

I had a pair of red shorts that were tight even after I had lost seventy pounds. When I reached my personal goal, those shorts slipped up and down with ease. Every time I put on those shorts, every time I spotted them, I remembered God's faithfulness. It was a token to remind me of His strength and prove His comfort.

The verse above indicates needing a token to prove to our enemies God's work in us, so that they would be ashamed. Enemies, perhaps, is a strong word, but prejudice against fat people prevails everywhere and no stronger anywhere than in the United States, where size indicates brilliance and competence. No person who has ever been overweight has been exempt from cruel taunts or discrimination in the workplace, school or church.

God's token of weight loss shows those people who hate (judge) us we are worthy. No longer do we hang our heads because our clothes are tight or we choose dessert. But, those *enemies* might be ashamed of their prejudice.

A token is for our enemies, but we need them, too.

Prayer: I hold to my token and give praise for Your faithfulness.

March 28

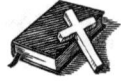

My Quiet Time is Essential

Be still, and know that I am God: I will be exalted among the heathen, I will be exalted in the earth. Psalms 46:10

Life hastens by with the speed of a roller coaster. Even good things like working for God can limit our time and tire our bodies. Our mental and physical health requires down time. We not only need plenty of sleep, but we need quiet time with our Creator.

Whenever we feel out of control, and want to eat everything in the refrigerator and pantry all in one sitting, take stock of what is going on in our lives.

Sometimes, finding the culprit is hard. No one had made me mad. My family was reasonably stable. I was well. Sometimes, the thing that was making me want to eat was simply a feeling that I'm overwhelmed. My husband often notices it first, and he'll say something like, "I thought you said you weren't going to do that Bible class this year?" Sometimes, he'll ask, "Why can't you just sit and talk with me? You keep scurrying around."

My answer to him might sound like, "I've got so much to get done by next week." In other words, I'm tired, bogged-down with *stuff*, and not dealing with life well. When I think about this, I realize that even though I'm getting sleep at night, I'm surrendering time to sit and talk with my Savior every day. Bingo. That's it. That's why I'm wanting to eat. Once again, my disease thrusts me into transplanting food into the place of God.

One time a friend told me, "Some say they're too busy to read the Bible and pray every day, but I say I'm too busy not to." That has become my creed. Are you troubled with food cravings? Check up on your quiet time.

Prayer: My quiet time is precious in Your sight, and mine.

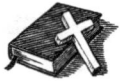

March 29

Junk Food

But I say unto you, That every idle word that men shall speak,
they shall give account thereof in the day of judgment.
Matthew 12:36

Candy and chips, cookies and donuts—junk food for the body. We label physical foods as junk when they do nothing to build up or give nutrition to our bodies. They, in fact, interfere with our digestion and increase weight that adds extra work to our heart and lungs. As computers infiltrated our world, the acronym "G.I.G.O." (Garbage In, Garbage, Out) focused our attention on the problem. Computers are only as good as what humans put in them. Our bodies function according to the nutrition we take into them.

Self put-downs and gossip, accusations and sarcasms—junk food from the mind. Jesus called these things "idle words." Mind junk foods reinforce the devil's work in our hearts and hamper God's healing from happening.

Overeaters give account for the idle words spoken out loud or to ourselves when we step on the scale and face up to weight gain or when we try to button our clothes without success.

Try **God's Junk**
> **J** oy
> **U** plifted heart
> **N** ew Life
> **K** id of the King

Prayer: Give me Your joy, uplifted heart, new life, and make
me a kid of the kingdom.

March 30

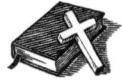

Giants Scare Me

And there we saw the giants, the sons of Anak, which come of the giants; and we were in our own sight as grasshoppers, and so we were in their sight. Numbers 13:33

When we want to lose weight, we may encounter giants, giants of:
1. Unbelief
2. Fear of failure
3. Fear of giving up something important to us
4. Fear of looking foolish
5. Disappointment

You might list other things, but when we look at our bloated bodies and remember the failures of our past, we view ourselves as tiny grasshoppers against the test before us.

Once a compulsive overeater, always a compulsive overeater. We are healed by depending on God's power one day at a time. When we drop His hand and rely on our abilities, we again face giants to relieve the compulsions in our lives. Once we've lost weight and walked with Christ, our giants might be:
1. Bad habits
2. Shame at retreating back into failure
3. Fear of what people will think of us after we've claimed victory
4. Again, unbelief

A man told Jesus. "I believe. Help thou my unbelief." Unbelief that we can do it, or do it again, looms giant-like.

Think of the giants keeping you from success. Just as the Israelites couldn't defeat the giants in their promised land, neither can we. Only God can slay the dragon, but only if we get out of His way.

Prayer: Lord, defeat the giants blocking my way to victory.

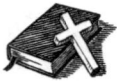

March 31

I Am Manipulative

Your attitude should be the kind that was shown us by Jesus Christ, who though he was God, did not demand and cling to his right as God, but laid aside his mighty power and glory; taking the disguise of a slave and becoming like men.
Philippians 2:5-7 Life Recovery Bible

As I began to heal, one thing the Holy Spirit pointed out to me was that I was manipulative. I didn't like that thought. I put myself into the martyr group of people. Woe is me. Manipulation nearly always involves selfishness. I suffered from low self-esteem. This seemed like an oxymoron.

Manipulation comes in several forms: pouting and crying, withdrawing approval, flattery, belittling others, dwelling on unequal treatment. God gives to each of us a will to do as we please. We can't control our mates, our children, our friends. They control themselves. Manipulation uses their love for us to get our own way.

Avoiding manipulation provides mental health and relief from compulsion. We do this by following Jesus' example and not demanding our own way, but being who we are, as God created us, some good, some bad, but definitely human, and also seeing others in the same light.

Prayer: Lord, destroy the selfish manipulation in my life.

April 1

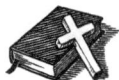

Examine Your Own Life

Examine yourselves, whether ye be in the faith; prove your own selves. Know ye not your own selves, how that Jesus Christ is in you, except ye be reprobates? 2 Corinthians 13:5

Anyone who follows Alcoholics Anonymous or Overeaters Anonymous or any of the twelve-step programs recognizes the need for a personal inventory. Paul urged in Corinthians to examine ourselves. This exhortation can be handled in many ways, but it's imperative that it be done to heal from any compulsive disorder or addiction.

Many books have been written to help us facilitate an inventory. I can only tell of my experience which worked well. The idea came from the Big Book of Alcoholics Anonymous.

I started in my childhood and followed through each phase of my life thinking of anyone who had angered me. Writing my inventory down brought reality to the process. My mind remembered it. I wrote how I was hurt when my parents pulled me away from my best friend, who I was angry at (my mother), how I handled it (I sulked), and what I was feeling (grief).

I wrote of a time when our good friend betrayed my husband in business. I wrote of a time I resented being left out when my daughter graduated from high school. Often, what I felt was resentment. As that book highlights, resentment is a killer. I can eat a kitchen full of food over resentment or envy.

Writing this inventory could take months, perhaps even years. After you finish, tear up those pages or burn them, or whatever it takes for you to mentally give them to God. Starting with a fresh slate fosters the healing process.

Prayer: Lord, bring to mind today anything that creates resentment, envy, grief, or anger.

91

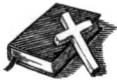

April 2

Making Amends Isn't for Wimps

Therefore if thou bring thy gift to the altar; and there rememberest that thy brother hath ought against thee; Leave there thy gift before the altar, and go thy way; first be reconciled to thy brother, and then come and offer thy gift.
Matthew 5:23,24

The Big Book of Alcoholics Anonymous lists twelve steps to recovery:

8. *Made a list of all persons we had harmed, and became willing to make amends to them all.*
9. *Made direct amends to such people wherever possible, except when to do so would injure them or others.*

Guilt brings inability to heal. Unable to go back and redo things or unsay unkind words, we're left with only one option: make amends. Usually we do this by apologizing. If we stole money or things, we should repay them. If we posted a hateful message on a social networking site, we should delete and post an apology. Whatever suits the wrong, we should do.

I first apologized to my long-suffering husband who bore the brunt of my angry words. After the apology, and with God's help, I treated him with more kindness. God enabled me to have a more even temper and less depression. I thank God for his ever-present assistance.

Next, I apologized to my daughters. All my family forgave me. Sometimes those to whom we make amends will refuse to forgive, but we must still do our part. After that, God can heal.

After our round of amends from the past, God expects us to watch for any slip-up or sin, so we may be quick to stop it and make amends before the hurt becomes a festering wound.

Prayer: Lord, help me be kind, and quickly let me know when I cause trouble, so I can apologize.

92

April 3

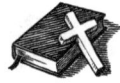

Blame Someone Else

And straightway in the morning the chief priests held a consultation with the elders and scribes and the whole council, and bound Jesus, and carried him away, and delivered him to Pilate. Mark 15:1

In Sunday school on Easter Sunday, the discussion brought out thoughts about the story of the crucifixion that I failed to notice.

The teacher asked the question about the verse above. "It was the religious leaders of the Jews that hated Jesus, not Rome, so why did they take him to Pilate?"

The usual answer was offered.

"Because the Jews couldn't give capital punishment."

Yes, that makes sense and could've been the foremost problem.

My son-in-law gave an answer that challenged my thinking. "Because they didn't want to take responsibility. They wanted the people to blame the Romans, who they disliked anyway."

I thought about that. How true. The blame game is innate in human nature. We desire to get our way, but we want to justify it and not take blame. We overeat of our own free will, then say all our family is overweight. It's in the genes. That may be true, but is that the true culprit? We might claim we couldn't get out of the party and the hostess made our favorite snack, as if she forced it down our throat.

Even Pilate knew the Jewish leaders' motivation. In verse 10 of Mark 15, it reads **"For he (Pilate) knew that the chief priests had delivered him (Jesus) for envy."** How many do we fool with our blame game? Certainly, not God.

Prayer: Lord, it's me standing in the need of help today. I can't blame anyone else.

93

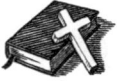

April 4

I Don't Give Up

We are pressed on every side by troubles, but not crushed and broken. We are perplexed because we don't know why things happen as they do, but we don't give up and quit.
2 Corinthians 4:8 Life Recovery Bible

I lived fifty of my years with despair. My mental attitude plagued my family with a multitude of fears and complaints. An emptiness filled my soul. At age fifty, I faced the realization that my physical health was deteriorating. What was left?

Christian friends assured me this wasn't sin. Gluttony and rebellion to eating as God desires is the one wrong condoned by the Christian community. More overweight people sit on the church pew than anywhere in the world.

If I wasn't sinning, but my eating controlled my life, then I must be crazy and hopeless.

The fact is: an overeating compulsion is:

1 ..A sin/rebellion to God
2. A disease with physical ramifications
3. Idolatry/putting food into the place of God
4. Lack of faith in God

Don't give up the fight. Give in to God. Just as if your sin was alcohol, adultery or drugs.

Prayer: Lord, I will not give up. I trust in You.

April 5

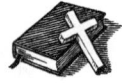

Paradoxes

But he said to me, My grace is sufficient for you, for my power is made perfect in weakness. 2 Corinthians 12:9 NIV

God's path to recovery exhibits many paradoxes.

I'm filled with amazement as I walk this way. God works in ways so far greater than man's. No man can understand.

When I am weak, I am strong.

When I am poor, I become rich.

When I give up control of my day, that day works out for my good.

When I confess powerlessness, I receive power.

When I give up, I gain control.

God's contradictions are man's relief. Trust Him and keep walking.

Prayer: Lord, I don't understand, but I have faith in You.

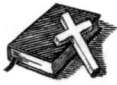

April 6

Give Blessings to God for His Purpose in You

... I am Joseph, your brother whom you sold into Egypt; But don't be angry with yourselves that you did this to me, for God did it! He sent me here ahead of you to preserve your lives.
Genesis 45: 4,5 Life Recovery Bible

When I began to recover emotionally, depression threatened to overwhelm me again because I realized the truth of my past actions. I remembered saying hurtful things to my young husband. My harsh words and actions brought sadness to my daughters over things they did because they were children. Friends and family thwarted my eating time or asked me to clean up messes when I had no energy. My resentment built over inconsequential things. Looking back over the years, I wept for the grief I'd caused, but like Joseph's brothers, I couldn't undo my wrongs.

Living in an attitude of gratitude to our Savior heals the wounds from our wrong-doing. Realizing God had a purpose in it all brings us to a lifetime of thankfulness.

I'm thankful that I never went into a deep sinful life as many alcoholics or drug addicts, but I might have been unable to pray with compassion for these without my own obsessive compulsion. Only reliance on God kept me from slipping off the edge of sanity. Total dependence on Him holds me steady when, even now, my feet teeter over the edge.

Our confidence in God allows us to believe in God's deliverance of others in need of His power, no matter how impossible the trial. God has it all under His control if we trust Him.

Prayer: Thank you, Lord, even for the bad times since it came all for Your purpose and plan.

April 7

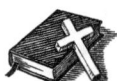

Pull Me Out of the Pit

... who redeems your life from the pit and crowns you with love and compassion. Psalms 103:4 NIV

"Oh, Lord, I hate myself. I hate my life. I'm a worthless piece of junk. I know stuffing food into my mouth is wrong, stupid and insane, but I can't stop. I feel I'm in a ditch. Life tantalizes me from above the ditch. I reach, but I can't touch that life. I am hopeless, useless and feel dead. Help me."

The above excerpt comes from one of my many journals. Writing has always been a release for me, a way of dumping my feelings while seeking solace. This was written on May 13, 1988. As you can tell, I was in the pit. God started my healing through the years of 1993 and 1994.

After God's healing, we still slip into the pit from time to time. Praise God, the slips become more shallow with each failure. We reach for God's strong arm. Sweat and blood drip from Jesus' brow as he tugs on us. Willingly, He sacrifices to redeem us from the pit. His actions and His words tell us, "You are loved. You are worth it."

Our eyes fill with tears as we remember the low times when Jesus saturated us with compassion and drew us to our knees in gratitude.

Prayer: All I can say today is thank you, Jesus.

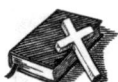

April 8

It's Not About the Food

Blind Pharisee! First clean the inside of the cup and dish, and then the outside also will be clean. Matthew 23:26 NIV

We look in the mirror and hate what we see. Someone makes a comment about our appearance and hurts our feelings. Then, we turn to a DIET. Yuck.

I hate diets. I started on the first one at age fourteen. I've succeeded at many kinds of diets. The only problem with every one of them was that "it's not about the food." If it was, a diet would be the answer. We'd curtail our food intake and lose weight. Problem solved.

Jesus gave advice to the religious leaders in His country during that time that they looked good on the outside, but the inside was corrupt.

A few years ago, that was my life. I would lose weight and look good on the outside. Compliments flowed, and sometimes I even worked in the field and gave talks on nutrition and weight loss because of my own accomplishments. Yet, inside, wounds festered, resentments churned, little rebellions fomented.

As with the Pharisees, we need to start on the inside. Ask Jesus to heal the wounds, destroy the resentments; and we need to submit the rebellions to Him. When we do that, the weight loss on the outside will take care of itself.

Prayer: Lord, clean my insides because my appetite reflects my corruption.

April 9

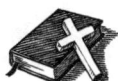

ABCs of Weight Loss

That if you confess with your mouth, "Jesus is Lord," and believe in your heart that God raised him from the dead, you will be saved. Romans 10:9 NIV

We Christians learn to witness and lead sinners to Christ by teaching them the ABCs of salvation.

A – Admit that you're a sinner.

B – Believe that God can deliver you from sin.

C – Confess that "Jesus is Lord" and has saved you.

These same ABCs follow with weight loss. Overeating falls into many categories; a disease, an addiction, a problem, and a sin. The sin of overeating (gluttony) can also follow the sin of idolatry (putting anything, in this case food, in the place of God). So, look at the ABCs of weight loss which are the first three steps of a twelve-step program for overeaters.

A – Admit that you're powerless over food.

B – Believe that God can overcome overeating in your life.

C – Confess that you're giving the problem to Jesus to handle.

Prayer: Lord, as I follow the ABCs of weight loss, I rely on You today.

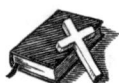

April 10

Cut Yourself Some Slack

As a father has compassion on his children, so the Lord has compassion on those who fear him; For he knows how we are formed, he remembers that we are dust. Psalms 103:13,14 NIV

As a parent, I trust my children over and beyond what anyone else might. I believe the best even when proven wrong. But, I beat myself up for the same thing.

Humans fail, but sometimes we succeed. That's true of us all. Someone caught in an addiction outwardly blames others but, inwardly, hates themselves.

We strive to remember that we're God's children. He knows where we came from and what experiences formed us into the people we are. Our trust in ourselves may be nil. Since we're His children, His compassion for us is great.

I will forgive anyone faster than I will forgive myself, but God's will demands I rely on God's assessment as my creator.

We are worthwhile because of how He made us—beautiful, useful people. We know, and God knows, we're not perfect but in Him we are exceptional.

Prayer: Lord, remind me of my worth in You especially when I do something stupid.

April 11

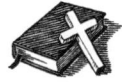

I Cried for Relief

When my spirit was overwhelmed within me, then thou knewest my path, in the way wherein I walked have they privily laid a snare for me. Psalms 142:3

At one time, I made the decision to teach a weight class at church. Plans were made to offer it on Tuesday night. My intentions were good, but I found that obligations on Tuesday and Wednesday nights each week taxed my time and sapped my energy. Though my intentions were good, I soon questioned if this was truly God's will. The group fell off and finally died in a few months time.

God knows our plans. He sees the snares set for us. We pray, but we hear our own selfish desires, not God's will. Even so, when our spirits become overwhelmed within us, we can call on God. Yes, God wants us to give Him our complaints and mistakes. We might as well tell Him. He knows anyway.

I would hope I wouldn't start something again without God in it, but I'm human and I might. Nevertheless, I can still call on Him.

Prayer: Show me Your way.

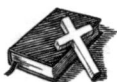

April 12

Stiff-Necked Won't Power

There is a way that seemeth right unto a man; but the end thereof are the ways of death. Proverbs 16:25

"You just need some will power," my husband and my mother both told me, time and time again. "Just push away from the table."

I tried but I couldn't do it, which reinforced my low self-esteem. Worldly wisdom advised me to get on a low calorie diet, or low fat, or low carbohydrate, and continue with it until I lost weight. I was told willpower is what helps me lose weight.

What my family and I didn't realize was that I had a strong unrelenting rebellious will that I used every day. My will power overcame every rational thought to say "I will to eat what I like, and I won't be controlled by anyone else in choosing what I eat." The craziness of this principle was that my will power overcame my conscious goals and desires. My invincible will power/won't power consumed my sanity and my life.

Will power isn't the answer. Will power can just as easily become won't power for an overeater. Only submitting our will to God's will gives us true healing from the driving force to eat more and eat wrong things.

Prayer: I submit to Your will now.

April 13

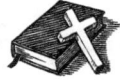

Patience, My Dear

*Knowing this, that the trying of your faith worketh patience.
But let patience have her perfect work, that ye may be perfect
and entire, wanting nothing. James 1:3,4*

I don't know about you, but I don't like to pray for patience.
When you do, you get trials. Of course, when you don't, you still
get trials because that is what builds faith and patience.

I used to rail at God for allowing me to gain weight and be a
person who can't stay away from food. I was angry that others
could eat whatever they wanted (it seemed like to me) and not
gain weight. Many times, I felt my burden was more than I
could bear.

Now, in looking back, I realize my burden was easy in
comparison, and I needed that plague to understand the addictive personality of others. Still, that compulsion drove me to
stick exactly with a diet. When I didn't lose quickly, my temper
exploded. When I lost slowly, my impatience grew.

Life overcoming a compulsion requires patience, always,
and faith in bucket loads, but the end result is worth the wait.

*Prayer: Okay, Lord, give me patience, so I can have a more
perfect, long-lasting healing.*

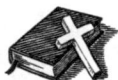

April 14

Get That Brain on the Right Track

And be not conformed to this world, but be ye transformed by the renewing of your mind, that ye may prove what is that good, and acceptable and perfect will of God. Romans 12:2

In the past, my husband and I were involved in multi-level marketing products. Our conferences and meetings were intended to inspire and encourage. Lots of the speakers talked about "stinking thinking." If we thought negative, we received the same. The Bible tells us we become what we think about. The battle for our minds rages onward whether we realize it or not.

Most of us have heard the story of the frog in the boiling pot of water. If we throw it in while it's boiling, the frog will quickly leap out, but if we put it in cool water and then heat it to boiling, it will die there. Movies, TV programs and commercial advertising know this. They hit us over and over until we become desensitized without even realizing it.

The next time we have these thoughts:

- I will always be fat.
- I've failed on so many diets, I know I'll never be able to stay on one.
- It's impossible for me.

Decide, is this really true right now or is it a mental CD we've played in our minds so many times that we believe it?

Start a new CD:

- I will soon be slimmer.
- I can not fail with Jesus with me.
- All things are possible with Him.

This will "transform your mind" for success.

Prayer: I believe for victory through You even in my eating.

April 15

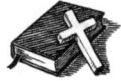

Contentment, an Illusive Trait

I know both how to be abased and I know how to abound every where and in all things; I am instructed both to be full and to be hungry, both to abound and to suffer need. Philippians 4:12

One of the single hardest things to do is to be content no matter what the circumstances. Overeaters must learn this trait to become an over-comer. Food is our drug of choice. We sedate ourselves when we're resentful or unhappy. We celebrate with it when we're elated.

What is wrong in our lives now? What is it we want to fix? Yes, we overeaters are fixers. The first time God brought this splashing into my face came with the separation of my daughter and son-in-law. Mom couldn't fix this, so I ate over it instead. Perhaps your husband has left, or you've lost your job, or you've been diagnosed with a chronic illness. Maybe you need to lose a hundred pounds.

Concentrate now on that thing that you must fix. Then, give up on it. Submit it to God. "Lord, I realize this may never happen. This is what I have to deal with at this point in life. I'll never lose those pounds. I can't have that job. My husband will not come back." Then, ask God for contentment, for His peace. He taught Paul to be content during terrible persecution. He'll get you through and bless you besides.

Prayer: Lord, bring forth Your peace in my life regardless of the circumstances.

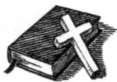

April 16

God is For Me

When I cry unto thee; then shall mine enemies turn back; this I know; for God is for me. Psalms 56:9

God listens when I cry out in disappointment.
God hears me when I scream out anger.
God cares when I feel disliked, mistreated.

As a compulsive overeater, at times I feel lonely and perse-cuted. Sometimes, in the midst of a crowd, I think I'm alone. No one really wants me or cares if I'm there. I'm not part of the group.

We cannot and must not entertain such thoughts, or we will overeat, and when we overeat, God cannot use our lives as He wishes. If we bow at the altar of good-tasting food or exhibit rebellion against eating what we think we should, we cease to be a tool for God.

Before you wallow in the next sinkhole:

- Stop.
- Think.
- Cry out.

God is always on our side.

Prayer: I need You today, Lord.

April 17

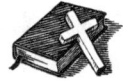

Taste Him

As newborn babes, desire the sincere milk of the word, that ye may grow thereby; If so be ye have tasted that the Lord is gracious. 1 Peter 2:2,3

My taste buds have been seared. For food to taste good, I need more sugar or more spice. No such food exists that's too sweet. The only secret to this is to train my taste buds to appreciate healthy foods without added sugar. God gave sweetness in the fruits and in some vegetables like sweet potatoes, corn, and butternut squash that he supplied.

The only way we like the sweetness created by God is if we leave off the sweetness manufactured by man. For several days, I refrained from eating sugar, and noticed an orange tasted sweet and delicious.

An example: My husband loves baked potatoes with everything on them—sour cream, butter, cheese, bacon. He must have butter. After suffering a stomach virus where he couldn't keep anything down, he began to add back more bland foods. He found he loved a plain baked potato with only a little salt.

If we haven't tasted God's sweetness or spiciness lately, we should leave off the fake stuff. Taste and see what God provides.

If you haven't read His word and feasted on God's banquet table lately, taste and see the sweetness of His communication.

Prayer: Lord, today I will taste Your word and Your provisions without additions.

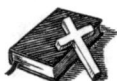

April 18

Stuffed, Yet Starved

Therefore thus saith the Lord God, Behold my servants shall eat, but ye shall be hungry; behold, my servants shall drink, but ye shall be thirsty; behold, my servants shall rejoice, but ye shall be ashamed. Isaiah 65:13

This prophecy comes to Judah describing those who refused to listen and obey God. But, wow, is it ever a picture of how I used to feel.

All God's servants or followers attended God's banquet table (usually at church). The food spread before us was intended to feed us, quench our thirst, and bring rejoicing in our hearts. But stuffed with food and sedated with sweets, I starved even in God's midst. Shame squelched the Spirit when I looked down at my bloated belly. I stood at God's fountain and felt parched.

Even though we enter the courts of praise and the gates of thanksgiving, the devil wins a victory if we are unable to partake. When we put God in His rightful place as king of our lives, we will no longer worship at the throne of Twinkies or bow at the altar of brownies. Think about it. What is your God? What do you wake up thinking about? If it's what you're going to eat first or where you can stop on the way to work to purchase goodies, you're starving.

Prayer: Today, I eat and drink of the Lord and rejoice in His keeping.

April 19

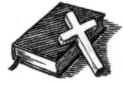

Dream On

For I know the plans I have for you, declares the Lord, plans to prosper you and not to harm you, plans to give you hope and a future. Jeremiah 29:11

Planning, dreaming, setting goals: these are good things for any individual. As compulsive overeaters, we quit dreaming. We quit hoping for something better. Along the way, we get lost in the food.

We awake in the morning thinking about what we will eat.

Instead, we should plan our goals or reach for our dreams.

When we were children, what did we want to be? Ballerinas, policemen, cowboys?

I wanted to be an airline hostess, then a singer, and—finally—a writer. But, year after year, I spent each day planning my next meal or snack. I spent a lot of thought on what I could sneak into my car, my purse, or a drawer to eat when I was by myself.

True example: I often made hot cinnamon rolls for my family. That's good, you think, except that I made twenty-four and ate eighteen of them. How did that help my family? Think of all the time on cooking them, eating them and cleaning up the mess, when I could've been living my dream and writing. What could I have accomplished with all that time?

Excessive food swallows our dreams.

EAT HEALTHY. DREAM ON.

Prayer: Lord, help me dream again.

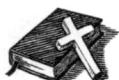

April 20

I'm Always Sick

... who forgives all your sins; and heals all your diseases.
Psalms 103:3

Let me state up front that I know there are exceptions, but when you're obese, disease strikes more often.

As a child, I fought asthma. When I was forty-five, it returned. My doctor treated me with medicine and breathing treatments and I improved, only to go around again a few weeks later. Certain foods, one of which is chocolate, causes asthma. Guess who couldn't stay away from Reese's?

Digestive trouble plagued me constantly. Alka-Seltzer or Tums held a permanent place among my medicines. Exercise would have helped many of my ailments, but at two hundred fifty pounds, I had no desire to move or move fast. I refused to give up fried food and sweets.

When I hit fifty, the doctor diagnosed me with high blood pressure, duodenum (digestive) inflammation, hiatal hernia and gall stones. I felt like I was falling apart.

Nightmare cases abound of people who have diabetes, heart problems, and other diseases brought on or complicated by obesity. When the doctor I worked for counted the risks for surgery, one of the main factors was weight.

I'm not saying that now I'm always well, but I do know I'm healthier now than I was seventeen years ago in an obese body. God heals our bodies, but notice that in the above verse, He connects sin and disease. He expects us to do our part. He'll do His.

Prayer: Help me eat healthier and exercise more and when I get sick, heal me.

April 21

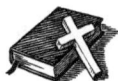

Make a Decision

Thou hast proved mine heart; thou hast visited me in the night; Thou hast tried me, and shall find nothing. I am purposed that my mouth shall not transgress. Psalms 17:3

Success can be as simple as making a decision. Ask God to take over your eating, decide on purchasing and planning healthy choices, then leave your food in His hands. Many things we do for God we do out of habit. Now, if that sounds wrong to you, hear me to conclusion.

With any addiction or compulsion, there is an element of habit involved. We turn to the same foods, the same friends, the same haunts that have tripped us before and made us fall. Salvation itself requires not only repentance for past wrongs, but asking Jesus to abide in our hearts. The devil loves empty vessels because he will enter and bring seven demons with him as in the Bible with the man called Legion.

I wanted to have a quiet time of prayer every morning, but time escaped me, and I couldn't do it. Finally, I set my alarm and decided to use the time before breakfast for prayer. At first, I fought rebellion against getting up early. I made a decision (or purposed in my heart) to pray every day. The more days I had done this, the more I never considered doing it otherwise, because I had set up a habit.

Make a decision to use your mouth for good, not evil. Your mouth can sin by speaking unkind or angry words, and your mouth can sin by taking in junk that bogs down your body like sludge in your car. Put legs to your decision. Buy healthy foods. Cook more. Pray a lot. Make a decision. Build a habit.

Prayer: I am purposed that my mouth not transgress.

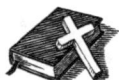

April 22

Don't Let Yourself Faint

He giveth power to the faint, and to them that have no might He increaseth strength. Isaiah 40:29

Eat sugar. Need more. Eat sugar. Blood sugar dips. Anyone who has ever experienced fluctuation of blood sugar knows how real it can be.

My middle daughter grew up loving fruits and disliking desserts. But she learned one thing about her mother. When Mom needed to eat, she better find food quickly. My daughter didn't understand it, but she knew the results. The first time she was pregnant and her body acted crazy, she had the same problem. She kept snacks in her drawer and refused to go long without eating. Suddenly, she understood Mom's problem. Eating simple carbohydrates causes dips in blood sugar requiring replenishment. Even if you've not had this problem, if you continue to eat improperly, you should watch for it.

Symptoms include:

- Fainting
- Dizzy
- Weak
- Nausea
- One bite of sugar helps

Sometimes, we eat healthy but don't rest properly. This can cause the same symptoms. Depression can also cause these health difficulties.

- Eat healthy.
- Sleep at night.
- Rest your mind during the workday.
- Move your body.
- Ask God for strength from fainting.

Prayer: Lord, I need Your strength to overcome fainting spells.

April 23

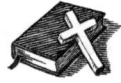

I Suffered Shame

And ye shall know that I am in the midst of Israel, and that I am the Lord your God, and none else; and my people shall never be ashamed. Joel 2:27

Thank you, Lord, for the unexpected benefits of losing weight. God answers prayer beyond what we anticipate or request. When we beseech God for help in losing weight, we don't know that what we need is a complete emotional healing.

Our outside reflects the turmoil inside. The battle rages in our minds first, but God heals all.

Two of the biggest heartaches of being grossly overweight are the looks of loathing and the derogatory comments. Most women who suffer a big mid-section have endured someone's insensitive question, "Are you expecting?" The pain is excruciating. Situations arise that hurt so much, they drive our eating underground, or to secret stashes.

A particularly shameful experience came to me in Amarillo, Texas. Our family was on vacation and stopped for lunch. The thoughtless hostess seated us in a narrow booth. I squeezed and pushed, but my huge body wouldn't fit. With haste, the manager rushed over with a chair to put on the end. My face burned. Tears streamed while half the restaurant watched. The food tasted like cardboard. Because of my shame, I survived only to get home and stuff my face in solitude.

God healed me so I never have to be ashamed again.

Prayer: Lord, in You, I am without shame and healed each day.

113

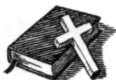

April 24

Get That Chip Off Your Shoulder

Love does not demand its own way, it is not irritable or touchy. It does not hold grudges and will hardly even notice when others do it wrong. 1 Corinthians 13:5 Life Recovery Bible

An overweight compulsive overeater bears a chip on his or her shoulder the size of Texas. We wait for someone to step on our toes, so we can cover our hurt with food. The thirteenth chapter of First Corinthians is known as the love chapter. Our goal should be to follow the standards set in that chapter, but our flesh fails. Most of us read the above words and think that the rules are impossible.

To reach for this kind of love involves first loving God then loving ourselves before we love others. The attainment of such perfection is in God's hands. We are inadequate for the task but require God's love in our hearts. At two hundred fifty pounds, I hated anyone with a slim body, anyone I considered perfect, compared to my imperfection.

When we stuff food in our mouths, we stuff hurt feelings, rejection and anger. When these emotions are healed, the chips fall off our shoulders because God replaces them with compassion.

Prayer: Lord, love others through me. Relieve me of touchy feelings.

April 25

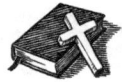

True Joy Is Possible

I have told you this so that my joy may be in you and that your joy may be complete. John 15:11 NIV

When we approach our journey toward weight loss, most of us prepare to suffer sacrifice.

Sacrifices include:

1. We give up the foods we love and going out to eat at restaurants we like.
2. We push our bodies to exercise when we desire mostly to sit and read.
3. We attend support meetings when we prefer doing other things.
4. Many times, we spend hard-earned money for clinics or groups that promise assistance in weight loss.

What we don't usually prepare for is the joys, the blessings, the extra benefits. When we turn to the Lord for our weight loss, we can prepare our minds for these:

1. Joy unspeakable, true and bountiful
2. Peace that passes all understanding
3. Healing for our soul, spirit and body
4. Energy to face tasks God gives us
5. Good foods to enjoy without guilt
6. No monetary outlay
7. Strength when we are weak.

Think not of the sacrifice, but dwell on the joy.

Prayer: Thank You, Lord, for all Your blessings on a weight loss journey.

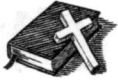

April 26

Free, At Last

For when we were controlled by the sinful nature, the sinful passions aroused by the law were at work in our bodies, so that we bore fruit for death. But, now by dying to what once bound us, we have been released from the law, so that we serve in the new way of the Spirit, and not in the old way of the written code. Romans 7:5-6 NIV

Diets don't work; freedom in Christ does. During the Old Testament times, the Israelites were given rules to follow. Priests made them rigid and uncompromising. Diets are that way. We're given foods we can eat and many that we can't eat.

A few years back, I lost a hundred and six pounds on a rigid diet of approximately eight hundred calories. The plan relied on a chemical reaction between foods, even one slip could set you back several days. I pursued it with diligence and won.

Happy about my victory, I purchased a franchise for that diet plan. But like with many diets I've done, eventually I introduced other foods into my eating and quickly gained. I fell prey to eating in secret so that I wouldn't ruin my business. By the time I put back all the weight, the headquarters took away my franchise—another failure in a dismal line of them.

Strict rules and regulations stir up our rebellious nature and bear the fruit of destruction. The early Christians found the freedom of Christ; so can we. When I came to Him and said, "I can't do it. I'm strong in many areas, but when it comes to food, I'm powerless. If You don't take over my eating, I'll keep gaining until I kill myself with food." What freedom to admit that I couldn't do it! What a release to lie back in Jesus' arms and wait for Him to work. He was always there, always able.

Prayer: Thank You, Lord, for today's freedom.

April 27

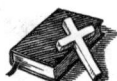

Benefits of Both Forward and Backward Thinking?

I thought about the former days, the years of long ago, I remembered my songs in the night. Psalms 77:5 NIV

Benefits of looking forward:

- We no longer listen to old tapes of how "lowly am I."
- We don't dwell on foods we can't handle.
- No regrets over past actions turned over to God.

Benefits of looking backward:

- We remember the pitfalls to avoid.
- We're thankful for how far we've come.
- When we think of food we used to like, we remember the harm it caused.

In our walk with the Lord in all areas of life, we receive blessing from both forward and backward thinking. God uses both. In the verse above, God used thinking of former days to bring back the memory of a song in the night. But, God also reminds us to forget the things that are past, and He will give us a new song.

Remembering old songs and singing new ones. Both are appropriate in their own way. Let God shine a light to our feet and a lamp to our path as we travel onward to liberty.

Prayer: Thank You for saving me from the past and guiding my future.

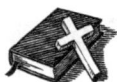

April 28

The Question Is

And when he was come into the house, the blind men came to him, and Jesus saith unto them; Believe ye that I am able to do this? They said unto him, Yea, Lord. Matthew 9:28

For years, I prayed "Lord, take away my craving for sweets and extra foods. Help me to lose weight and eat normally." Then I left the altar, picked up my problem again, and over-ate when I left the church.

What was the difference nineteen years ago when I started losing and never stopped until I chose to stop? What's the difference that gave me a sincere desire to eat healthy, exercise, and do God's will?

The difference is the answer to one question. It's the same question Jesus often asked in His earthly ministry. The same question he asked the blind men seeking healing in the verse above.

Do you believe I am able to do this?
Do you believe I can stop your compulsion?
Do you believe I'll be faithful to help when you call?
Faith unlocks the door to healing.
Do you really believe?
If not, first ask for help to believe. That's the key.

Prayer: Lord, I believe. Help my unbelief today.

April 29

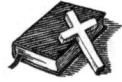

Help, My Youth is Gone

Who satisfieth thy mouth with good things; so that thy youth is renewed like the eagles. Psalms 103:5

We may feel that we sacrificed our youth being overweight, and it makes us angry. A fountain of youth flees our grasp so quickly. We can't do a remake of our younger years, but the next best thing comes from the Lord.

Only the Lord can bring satisfaction with the food we eat. Only the Lord can renew the energy we lost from extra poundage. Only the Lord can make us soar like an eagle, finding new hope and new joy at an older age.

Get over the guilt.
Give up the anger.
Trust in your new beginning.
Trust in your future with God.

Prayer: Lord, renew what I have lost through my compulsion.

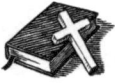

April 30

Choose Happiness

This day I call heaven and earth as witnesses against you; that I have set before you life and death; blessings and curses. Now choose life, so that you and your children may live and that you may love the Lord your God. Deuteronomy 30:19 NIV

Snow and ice kept me shut in the house for days causing my husband and me to get irritable and sharp with each other because of boredom and the inability to get in the car when we wanted. I suffered from lack of independence, too much togetherness, and nothing to do. My husband's sharp retort to my trying to control his space angered me. For the rest of the day, we circled around each other with a wide berth and spoke infrequently. I prayed and apologized, but his reply made me mad again.

By the second day, I couldn't stand it anymore. I told him "I don't like being mad at you." He said "then don't." He meant it to be cute, but his words held much wisdom.

Our attitude is our choice, just like the Israelites who could choose blessings or curses. No one can make us be angry or sad or downhearted. We do that to ourselves.

During the days of overeating, depression and self-condemnation were constant allies. A bad mood could send me to the kitchen or the store for more or sweeter treats. Cyclical in nature, I then over-ate and became more depressed. I ate and was eaten up with guilt and internal rage.

I took my husband's advice that day. I quit being angry at him, and the day improved. God illumined the way to changing my attitude. Only through His power can we accomplish the reversal.

Prayer: Thank You, Jesus, for helping me choose happiness today.

May 1

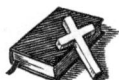

Eat with Me

Here I am: I stand at the door and knock. If anyone hears my voice and opens the door, I will come in and eat with him, and he with me. Revelation 3:20 NIV

What a promise. Think of Jesus sitting across the table every time you sit to eat. Now, think of Him sitting by your side while you stuff candy in your mouth faster than you can swallow. If you ask Jesus into your heart and life, but continue to overeat, you produce this despicable scene.

However, if you let Jesus control what you eat, you can have true communion.

Your meals can be a time of –

Replenishment
Regrouping
Rejoicing
Recovery
Reducing
Reflection
Refreshment
Reliance
Relaxing

Think of eating in this context. Think of it like prayer, a time to give God honor for what He's done and what He's going to do. A time set aside by God to renew our energy and strength to serve Him. Now, what sounds best—a healthy balanced meal or a sack of donuts?

Prayer: Today, make my meals and snacks a new way of worshiping and fellowshipping with You.

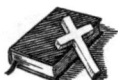

May 2

Wanted: Students and Teachers

"I want to make the simpleminded wise!" he said. "I want to warn young men about some problems they will face. I want those already wise to become the wiser and become leaders by exploring the depths of meaning in these nuggets of truth." Proverbs 1:4-6 New Recovery Bible

For many years, heartache and desperation designed much of my world because of an addiction I could not control. I gave my heart to Jesus at an early age. I believed in divine healing. The deeper the hole I dug for myself, the more I realized my addiction was rebellion toward God.

God led His people, the Israelites, out of Egypt and into the promised land, but in times of rebellion, he left them to their chosen fates until they called out to Him. When they did, He answered and saved them. But His people, just like me, couldn't leave it in God's hands.

God leads us out of Egypt (overeating), but if we refuse to give up treats we fight for independence from God. As capable strong-willed people, we feel we should be able to choose what we want to eat. We think we can control this disorder. But we can't.

God teaches us from His Holy Word so that young people, if they listen and submit, could bypass the heartaches of sin. we see young people today with the same problem we have who are going on one diet after another and not leaving it in God's hands.

I pray the word makes ones like myself wiser and willing to teach the younger. God uses we older rebels to be leaders.

Where are you on the journey? Younger needing teaching, or a teacher needing to be strong and lead the way?

Prayer: Lord, make me wise to lead. Keep me on Your course.

May 3

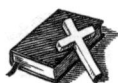

God's Peace

If you do this, you will experience God's peace, which is far more wonderful than the human mind can understand. His peace will keep your thoughts and your hearts quiet and at rest as you trust in Christ Jesus. Philippians 4:7 New Recovery Bible

Recovery is a process. Many times we live for years in denial. We want freedom to do what we prefer. Because we're adults and work hard, we think we should control our own destiny—with God's help, of course.

That's the way I felt. I had freedom. I ate what I wanted; donuts in the morning at work and Reese's candy stashed to eat whenever I was home and no one was watching. Yeah, I controlled my destiny alright.

But I had no peace.

God's peace is worth whatever we have to pay.

For me, I had to give up forever some treats I loved. I had to give up the concept that I was free to do as I pleased. Anything I decided to eat, I had to eat while others watched. I had to stop being secretive.

God's peace keeps your heart at rest. We don't know how to accept it and utilize it but, through the recovery time, God teaches us. Give up the freedom. Reach for the peace.

Prayer: Teach me what I need to learn about Your peace today.

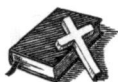

May 4

How Much Do You Think About Food?

Therefore take no thought, saying, What shall we eat? Or What shall we drink? Or Wherewithal shall we be clothed?
Matthew 6:31

Most compulsive overeaters think about food all the time. It's a constant struggle.

When the compulsion, instead of God, ruled my life, if you had asked me how much I thought about food I would have said "Always." After the morning donuts were halfway digested, I planned lunch. With the last bite of my McDonald's hamburger, I thought of going by the store for treats on the way home from work. "Always." Food controlled when I did things and why I did not do things.

God wants us to be so in love with Him that we think about Him "always." As the Bible tells us, we can't serve two masters. Neither can our minds rest on two thoughts at the same time.

In this verse, God reminds us to not dwell on the temporal, what we eat, drink, or wear, but to put first His kingdom. In other words, think on God and His goodness and faithfulness and provision, "always."

Prayer: Lord, keep my mind stayed on You and food in its proper place as sustenance.

May 5

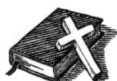

A Different Viewpoint

Therefore if any man be in Christ, he is a new creature, old things are passed away; behold all things are become new.
2 Corinthians 5:17

Every time I started a new diet, I prepared my mind. I concentrated on positive input. "I can do this. I've not tried this diet. This plan makes better sense than the others. With the pills or shots, I won't be hungry this time."

This time –

This diet –

These helps –

This support group –

Always I focused on changing my mind or thought patterns. But God looks on the whole person, and He made us soul, spirit and body after His image.

Losing weight requires not just a better mindset, but a totally new way of looking at food. God provided food as nourishment for our physical body. He never intended it to feed our mental or spiritual needs. No matter how much good-tasting food we stuff into our pie hole, only God can fill the hole in our hearts.

Don't think of it as positive outlook.

Think of it as letting your entire being fall back into God's trustworthy arms.

Prayer: Let me see life and food through Your eyes.

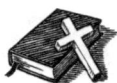

May 6

Get Me Out of Prison

Set me free from my prison, that I may praise your name.
Psalms 142:7 NIV

Once upon a time, I claimed my freedom to do whatever I pleased. To eat whatever I wanted. I was a responsible adult. No one should tell me I can't eat something. That was unacceptable, and I refused to succumb to that philosophy. I merely needed to exercise more self control to stay away from food that made me fat, sluggish and unhealthy.

My freedom imprisoned my spirit. I slid into the depths of depression. My life filled with emptiness no matter how many sweet-tasting delicacies I ate.

God prepared a place in each of our hearts that can only be filled by Him. That was His intention—we would long for God in our lives, and we would turn to Him in worship. But, when we try to fill that hole with other things, or other people, or other gods, we build prison walls around our spirit too strong to break.

Don't let anyone tell you otherwise. If you overeat compulsively and think of food twenty-four hours a day, you've got a spiritual problem. I'm not saying you may not be saved and going to heaven, but your spirit is dry and brittle, your soul in jail.

Prayer: Lord, break down every prison wall I build for myself.
Freedom only comes through You.

May 7

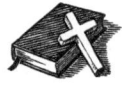

My Faith is Weak

And Jesus said unto them, Because of your unbelief, for verily, I say unto you, If ye have faith as a gram of mustard seed, ye shall say unto this mountain. Remove hence to yonder place, and it shall remove and nothing shall be impossible unto you. Howbeit this kind goeth not but by prayer and fasting. Matthew 17:20

A mustard seed is so small we almost need a microscope to see it at all. Holding one reminds us of how weak faith can be magnified if placed in the Master's hand.

Power in positive thinking can be real, but all the thought processes we utilize to increase our faith are few. However, we shouldn't let this discourage us.

First, act as if your hopes have been realized. Choose low fat, complex carbohydrates and lean protein at the store. Plan your meals for the day. Read and dwell on positive reinforcement. Yet, all this is nothing unless you rest in His power. Pray and fast. That's Jesus' instructions for difficult circumstances.

You see, I know I can't stick with that plan indefinitely.

I know my positive thinking is as a mustard seed of faith.

I know my weakness.

I know God's power.

Give Him your mustard seed of faith, and He will move the mountain of failure from your life.

Prayer: Lord, my faith is small, so I rely solely on You.

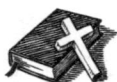

May 8

Green-Eyed Monster

For jealousy is the rage of a man; therefore he will not spare in the day of vengeance. He will not regard any ransom; neither will he rest content though thou givest many gifts. Proverbs 6: 34,35

Jealousy equals rage. Contentment eludes anyone filled with jealousy. Our English slang for this emotion is the green-eyed monster termed from the clichéd type of jealousy, a woman with green eyes and red hair. Monster explains how the rage transforms a person into an unbelievably demon-like persona.

No inciting event is required for jealousy to rear its ugly head. Many times, our perception of that event is enough. To explain that, here's an example from my own life from a few years ago. For healing, I wrote about it in my journal.

What actually happened:

My mother-in-law complimented someone else, saying she needed help so much and was thankful to that person for supplying it.

How I perceived that event:

My mother-in-law had berated me because I had not done enough, but *this person* had done a lot less, so I was jealous of her and angry at my mother-in-law.

Fill in the blanks for your own example. We all have them, but overeaters use them as an excuse. That green-eyed monster is a killer for compulsive people.

What do you do with those feelings of jealousy? Give them to Jesus. Ask Him to change them, throw them away, replace them with love. That's our only options or else we eat, and eat, and eat.

Prayer: Heal any feelings of jealousy I might have today.

May 9

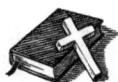

It's Been a Bad Day

My God is my rock, in whom I take refuge, my shield and the horn of my salvation. He is my stronghold, my refuge and my savior—from violent men you save me. 2 Samuel 22:3 NIV

I wish I didn't ever have a bad day.

I wish God kept those times from happening.

The fact is; we live in a sinful world. The devil is the prince of this world. God allows him a measure of freedom until God says it's enough. Until that time, the devil plagues us and, some days, we don't possess energy to battle.

That's what I call a bad day.

But, when I'm weak –

Yes, God is strong.

When I'm poor –

God is rich.

When I'm needy –

God owns the oil, gold and precious metals in the world and beyond.

When my feet slip –

He is my rock, my stronghold, my refuge.

Prayer: Thank You, Jesus, when my day is bad, You are enough.

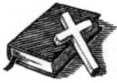

May 10

Wonders from God

Call unto me, and I will answer thee, and shew thee great and mighty things, which thou knowest not. Jeremiah 33:3

Jeremiah stood faithful to God though many around him doubted, disobeyed, and fell. Judah's king, Zedekiah, desired good news of victory, but he worshipped his idols and refused to stay true to God.

Many times, friends will start on the path to dependence on God for weight loss but give up because it's too hard. A friend of mine was like King Zedekiah. She only wanted victory on the scale and refused to accept the ups and downs of recovery.

Jeremiah prophesied, as God instructed him to do, that the Chaldeans would overwhelm Jerusalem, and Zedekiah would be taken prisoner. Jeremiah depended on God. Zedekiah imprisoned Jeremiah because of his words. It was a hard time for the prophet.

When my friend and I both showed gains for two weeks in a row, she quit. I suggested a special prayer time together, but that didn't fit into what she wanted to do. I fasted and prayed.

God spoke to Jeremiah in the above verse while he was yet in prison. God can speak to us when we feel like we're in prison—when we're discouraged with results. He promises to show us great and mighty things.

The losses started for me once more. I lost ninety-five pounds—a great and mighty thing to one who had failed so much. My friend is still heavy.

Prayer: I call on You today and know You can work wonders on my behalf.

May 11

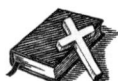

No Comparisons, Please

You shall not covet your neighbor's house. You shall not covet your neighbor's wife, or his manservant or maidservant, his ox or donkey or anything that belongs to your neighbor.
Exodus 20:17 NIV

I might add, "Thou shall not covet thy friend's body or beauty."

God thought coveting (envying) so important that He listed it as one of His Ten Commandments for the people of Israel. Envy can kill our ability to be who God created us to be. Envy hinders our prayers, damages our witness, and destroys our weight loss efforts.

A few years ago, I would've said I don't envy anyone. I wouldn't have been lying. I truly thought I didn't, but God convicted me. I suffered stiff movements, tied tongue and feelings of intimidation every time I was around one certain lady in my church.

She was about my age and absolutely perfect. Every hair was in place, her makeup exact, her clothes from designer shops I couldn't afford. And her figure—shapely without an ounce of fat, curves in all the right places. I was sure she didn't know how to have fun, or she would mess up her hair, but soon I found her to be witty, sweet and able to laugh at herself.

I argued I didn't envy her. I regretted that I was ugly and fat. I wished I could be more like her, but I wasn't. I was fat.

Comparison to others is coveting, envying. It's sin. In this, we disobey God by calling what He has created as ugly. Until I prayed for God to rid me of covetousness, I could not heal.

Prayer: Lord, deliver me from comparisons today.

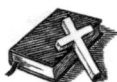

May 12

Different Tallow Trees

There are different kinds of gifts, but the same Spirit; there are different kinds of service, but the same Lord. There are different kinds of working, but the same God works all of them to all men.
1 Corinthians 12:4-6 NIV

In our back yard, about ten years ago, my husband planted two Chinese tallow trees.

One grew quickly and gave good shade within two years, and in the fall, its leaves provided brilliant color. The other was scrawny and sparse, and its colors weren't as bright.

Through their life span, they have differed. The bigger one stopped growing and gave little color. Berries grew thick and unique. The smaller one became the larger, fuller tree with the most brilliant color.

Now, ten years later, the faster-growing tree remains small, with lots of berries, and shows muted color. It sheds its leaves with the first cold wind.

The slower-growing tree is large and shades our patio swing in the summer. But, it never gave berries and it never turns colors. It sheds leaves only when the new growth comes in the spring.

Different, but equally of value. One for berries and color, the other for its shade.

God made us the same way. To lose weight and gain self value, we have to praise God for who He made us—different but equally of value to Him.

Prayer: Lord, use me today however You want.

May 13

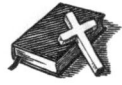

Commitment

Commit your way to the Lord; trust in Him. and He will do this: He will make your righteousness shine like the dawn. The justice of your cause like the noonday sun. Psalms 37:5-6 NIV

Commit—according to the dictionary, it means entrust, charge, or consign.

Look at the word consign. That reminds me of the second-hand shops in my hometown. It's the latest rage, and women love them. When I lost ninety-five pounds, I had a closet full of clothes that were too big. I loved having the problem but didn't have the solution. One of my friends had an overweight daughter. She came and picked out a few favorites.

I took the rest of my BIG clothes to a consignment shop. I left them in the store owner's care to use as merchandise for her clients. Any she sold, she gave a percentage (a blessing) of that purchase amount to me. That's what I think of when I see the word consign.

We consign our lives to Jesus. He uses it as He desires for His kingdom (store). We reap a percentage (benefits/blessings) with each time His kingdom advances.

Have you given your life into God's consignment?

Prayer: Lord, my blessing and my mission are in Your hands to use.

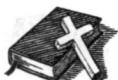

May 14

Forget About It

For I will forgive their wickedness and will remember their sins no more. Hebrews 8:12 NIV

When I pull into my garage after going to the grocery store, I love to spot my husband's car at home because I know he can lift my burden of groceries and bring them into the house, relieving me of that weight. Once I told him to pile everything on the sofa so it wouldn't be on the kitchen counter where I needed to start dinner. Unfortunately, he didn't follow my instructions. By habit, he placed every sack on the kitchen counter.

I huffed, puffed, and transferred every item from the counter to the sofa struggling against the weight of five pounds of flour and two milk cartons. When I'd finished, my back ached from the heavy lifting, and my anger fomented against my husband.

"Why didn't you remind me?" he asked. "I meant to lift them for you."

Are we like that with God? Do we ask for our sins to be removed, but then pick them up again to carry?

Satan uses past sins to disable our effectiveness. When I repented and asked Jesus into my heart, He took my burden of sin and cast it as the Bible says, "as far as the east is from the west." Therefore, I can be sure that any condemnation I have over sins from my past comes from the devil.

Leave them with Jesus. Talk to him about any anguish you feel. He means to relieve us of those burdens. Not unlike unwanted pounds on our bodies, resentment and anger are too heavy for us to bear.

Prayer: Lord, I leave my sins at Your feet. Help me to forget about them as You have done.

May 15

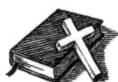

Planning, Patience, and Perseverance

Wherefore seeing we also are compassed about with so great a cloud of witnesses, let us lay aside every weight, and the sin which doth so easily beset us, and let us run with patience the race that is set before us. Hebrews 12:1

When she was in fifth grade, our middle daughter amazed us with her determination to win one of her school's field day activities. She chose the flex arm hang. Understand that this girl weighed about fifty pounds and when her scrawny arms tensed, they resembled two pencils with lumps of clay. She entered the event. She chose a direction. She practiced her skill.

By mid-morning of field day, competitors stood in line. Two kids at a time grabbed hold of the bar and held on while teachers timed them. When my daughter's challenge came, murmurs rose. Not too many gave her much encouragement. With muscular arms, her partner flexed and held, while my daughter's arms remained tense, her face set in a deep scrunch.

Finally, the partner dropped from exhaustion. Shouts rang out. "Give up, honey." Sweat ran down my daughter's hairline and dripped to the ground, but she refused to stop. By the time her feet touched the ground, she had nothing left—nothing but the admiration of everyone watching.

Once we decide to follow the Lord in the way we eat, we choose the "race set before us." Entering the track meet or the field day requires the three Ps. We must **Plan** (practice), have **Patience** (weight loss success doesn't come quickly) and **Perseverance** (we don't give up when the going gets tough).

Prayer: I've entered the race. Guide my steps, today, Lord.

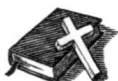

May 16

My Gigantic Guilt Complex

Therefore, there is now no condemnation for those who are in Christ Jesus. Romans 8:1 NIV

My husband tells me I have the biggest guilt complex of anyone he knows. Any bad thing that happens is somehow my fault. Sometimes I lie sleepless at night over words I've said but didn't feel like they sounded right, or words I didn't say that I feel I should have.

My children or grandchildren do wrong—I carry the blame.

Our church has a need for volunteers in a particular area—I should do it despite the fact that I'm already doing what God directed me to do.

I miss church because I'm exhausted—I've let down everyone in our church.

A group falters then folds—I didn't do enough even if it's not my responsibility.

Can I hear an Amen?

The Holy Spirit issues conviction to our minds to nudge us into what He desires. But, if we walk with Christ and lean on Him, any guilty conscience (condemnation) comes from the devil. God tells us to resist the devil. Refuse to carry that load. Ask Jesus to lift it from your shoulders.

If you over-ate today or ate a food that you should stay away from, ask Jesus to relieve the guilt. Walk in victory knowing, though it may be unseen, it's just ahead.

Prayer: Lord, help me walk without condemnation today.

May 17

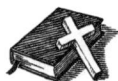

There's Power in Our Words

For in many things we offend all. If any man offend not in word, the same is a perfect man, and able also to bridle the whole body. James 3:2

What word do you use when you think of weight loss?

D – Deprivation
I – Intimidating
E – Eating rules
T – Torment

Instead, think of uplifting words. As the verse above tells us, we all offend with our words. Sometimes, we offend ourselves, and power rests in our words, in our viewpoint.

W – Wholesome
H – Healthy
O – Optimistic
L – Light and Lively
E – Energetic

The words we use do make a difference in our approach to the challenge. Swear off diets. Decide to live wholly.

Prayer: Lord, give me Your word to apply to my problem today.

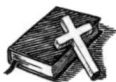

May 18

True Humility

Humble yourselves before the Lord, and He will lift you up.
James 4:10 NIV

In my "fat" days, I ran myself down and thought of myself as ugly and worthless, so when I was told I would be unsuccessful at God's weight loss plan without humility, I tuned out their words. Who was more humble than I?

My Super Thesaurus gives synonyms for the word humility as unpretentious, quietness, lack of pride.

What humility is not: It's not low self-esteem.

Stories abound in the Bible telling us how much God loves us. He created us perfect in His eyes. How do you think it makes Him feel when we demoralize or crush someone He created and blessed?

Think of the words the thesaurus lists:

Unpretentious or not trying to be something we're not.

Quietness—not boastful, arrogant or unbending.

Lack of pride—God hates pride. It's one of the sins He lists as hurtful. He doesn't mean the gratitude we should feel for the shapely legs or vibrant hair or good conversational skills. He means thinking more highly of ourselves than we ought to think.

Pride runs down others.

Low self-esteem runs down ourselves.

God wants us to live in an attitude of gratitude to God for what He's given us and done for us. If we act with humility, God uses us for His kingdom. He lifts us up and makes us great.

Prayer: Lord, teach me true humility, not pride, not self abasement.

May 19

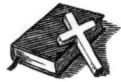

Is A Strong Will Pride?

Pride goeth before destruction and an haughty spirit before a fall.
Proverbs 16:18

A human spirit is a mighty giant
In fragile, soft disguise.
Life hurls pellets at its head
Hits stomach, groin, and eyes.

The world poises a hefty stance
And blows arrows to the heart
That mighty spirit wobbles, shakes.
It jerks and rips apart.

But as you watch, the giant sits up.
He gathers his scattered sections.
He stands up proud with head held high
Tougher than all detection.

Again the giant is hit with rocks.
He tumbles and falls to the ground.
Evil laughs at the wounded giant
Parts strewn across the land.

He's dead this time, says evil's helper.
He will never rise again,
But out of the trash heap of despair
We see a clutching hand.
Janet K. Brown

Prayer: Let my strong human spirit fall in submission to
Your sovereignty.

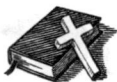

May 20

At the End of Yourself

They reeled and staggered like drunken men; they were at their wit's end. Then they cried out to the Lord in their trouble, and He brought them out of their distress. Psalms 107: 27,28 NIV

Machines and appliances are less than my forte. My can opener quit cutting properly. I struggled and worked and wore myself out trying to MAKE it to do what I wanted. My husband took it from my hands, set it on the counter, put the can directly under the magnet and mashed the button. My can of tomatoes swung around and dropped, opened. What a difference when put into the hand of one more adept at handling mechanical things.

Just like my life—more functional when in the hands of the One who knows how to make it work. Why do I not release it before I struggle, fume and reach "my wit's end?"

Different people touch bottom at different places. My bottom came in January, 1993. I had tried everything I knew, but obesity had me conquered. The devil held his foot to my mid-section and counted the beats to my destruction.

I entered the back room of my church. Our music minister, who was overweight himself, rose to the podium and said, "If you're ready to give up the fight, you're in the right place." I thought he was crazy, or else I was. The latter was correct. With every ounce of strength I possessed, I fought the obesity battle. I was ready to give up "my will power," my control.

Have you put your life into the Master's Hand?

Prayer: You are the master. Control my life today.

May 21

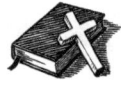

Rebel Without A Prayer

Some became fools through their rebellious ways and suffered affliction because of the iniquities. Psalms 107:17 NIV

I remember my first act of rebellion. In my photo collection, I have a picture of a four-year-old girl in a white sweater and a white pleated skirt. I looked sweet, but that day my sinful nature made itself known and caused my first spanking. All over the house, I strewed my father's Sunday newspaper.

He stared at me. "Pick it up."

My chin lifted in determination. "No."

Dad told me several times.

I refused.

"Pick them up, or I'll spank you."

With the strongest will a four-year-old could muster, I said, "No."

My dad swatted my legs with his belt until the skin broke.

I picked them up, then later bragged to my friends that my dad spanked me until I bled. I played the martyr.

After I left the control of my earthly father, my rebellion sprang up in adulthood toward my heavenly father. When first convicted of this, I failed to see the sin. At age seven, I had asked God into my heart. But in college, I drew away from God. Later, I returned to Him with humility. I attended church, taught Sunday school, and attempted to please God.

In the realm of eating—our resentments, playing the role of martyr—our childhood rebellion may remain. We suffer agony and emptiness because of sin.

When God began His healing on me, He reminded me of the incident at the age of four. I never outgrew that rebellious child, stomping my foot at God and saying "No."

Prayer: Help me say yes to You, Lord, whatever You ask of me.

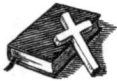

May 22

By Your Words

For by your words you will be acquitted, and by your words you will be condemned. Matthew 12:37 NIV

Besides God, who hears all the words we say?

Us.

In the throes of my addiction, I once yelled at my young husband some hateful words. Long ago, he forgave me. But in my lowest time, I recall those words and wish I could retrieve them.

God tells us that our words will acquit or condemn us. The definition of acquit is to release or clear one from a responsibility or charge. Loving words free our spirit, lighten our mood and improve our testimony.

I bear a heavy load of condemnation when my words hurt or cause pain. Peace leaves. Misery remains. God can heal that pain, but He warns us to watch our words. To stay free of our addictions or compulsions, we must steer around wrecks from our speech. Be slow to speak. Pray for help before your tongue slips.

Prayer: Help me watch my words today.

May 23

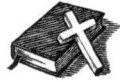

It's A Matter of Trust

The Lord himself goes before you, and will be with you: He will never leave you nor forsake you. Do not be afraid; do not be discouraged. Deuteronomy 31:8 NIV

Our middle daughter was a daddy's girl. While we vacationed when she was about two, we stayed at a hotel with a swimming pool. My husband and older daughter swam. My youngest and I reclined in a lounge chair. I watched the middle girl step to the edge of the pool. I called to her, but she ignored me.

"Dad," she called and proceeded to jump into ten feet of water.

My husband rushed to the spot and quickly retrieved her. Shaking the water from her hair as she came up for air, my two-year-old adventurer giggled. She trusted her father to handle the situation.

Nothing in our lives takes our Father God by surprise. It's a matter of whether or not we trust Him to keep us safe.

After we embark on a healthy, common sense weight loss plan, we must trust Him to guide us through the rough times, direct us through challenging rapids, and stand up for us when our desires fail.

It's a matter of trusting God.

Prayer: Lord, I trust and rely on You to increase my trust quotient.

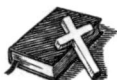

May 24

Celebrate Your Success

O Lord, the king rejoices in your strength. How great is his joy in the victories you give! Psalms 21:1 NIV

A weight loss journey begins with the first step and continues down the path, one stepping stone at a time.

When I began, failure loomed in my mind like a formidable barrier. I forgot every victory and remembered only lapses. Doing this hindered my progress. Our music minister, who led our weight class, urged us to forget failures and dwell on our accomplishments. My life was a mess. Counting good things went contrary to my instincts, but the more I tried, the easier it became.

When I confessed to my friend how I'd fallen on my face and ate everything in sight, he asked "So, how many days did you eat well, before this day?"

"Thirteen," I said.

He looked at me with disbelief. "Did you reward yourself for the thirteen days?"

I shook my head.

"Then you have no right to berate yourself for this day."

The verse above tells us God takes great joy in our victory. How can we do less?

Prayer: Thank You for my triumph yesterday.

May 25

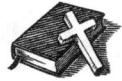

I'm Teetering

Free me from the trap that is set for me, for you are my refuge.
Psalms 31:4 NIV

Statistics tell us that a church can be the most dangerous place for one who has a problem with food. In trying to stay away from the very appearance of evil, Christians can come up with a long list of things not to do. All believe we should avoid drug addiction, many avoid alcohol, most stay away from nicotine, and many denominations shy away from movies or dancing. Young Christians often cry out, "What can we do?"

Everyone requires food to live. Ah, one thing we can all agree on, whether Christian or not. Fun times around a church group focuses on food—potlucks, dinner on the ground, Christmas parties.

Christians appear to bless the addiction to food as acceptable. Therefore, some of the biggest traps set for us come from inside the church building or meeting with a group from church. Temptation lurks at most parties, meetings or fellowships.

Could that be what David understood when he cried out to God in the above verse? Perhaps not. But, we compulsive overeaters of the twenty-first century face unsurpassed temptation in this area. To start a weight loss class in church elicits jokes and taunts. Few understand the reality of the problem.

God understands.

He is the overeaters' refuge.

You are not alone. Try suggesting, and helping to supply, healthier options. When faced with a trap, call on Jesus to guide you through the land mine.

Prayer: Guide me around the temptations at my church.

145

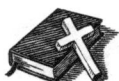

May 26

Two Commandments

This is the first and greatest commandment; And the second is like it; Love your neighbor as yourself. Matthew 22:38,39 NIV

In the Old Testament, God gave the Israelites ten commandments. Jesus condensed them into two. Love God and love your neighbor. Years ago, I thought I did this, but was I ever wrong.

Notice the way Jesus framed the command: Love your neighbor AS YOURSELF. If I had loved my neighbors as myself, I would have hated them because I hated myself. What a slap in the face to my Creator.

First, we must learn to love ourselves. Then, and only then, can we love others. To receive true healing in this area, we should turn the commandment backwards and do a mental check.

Other people make mistakes, but I'm quick to forgive. Check.

I believe the good in people. Check

I'm optimistic that others will do the right thing. Check

I make positive comments toward others, since I'm conscious of the power of my words. Check

Can we improve? Can we say the same things about ourselves?

Prayer: Today, I determine to love God, myself, and others—in that order.

May 27

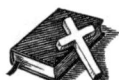

Secrets are Killers

Stolen waters are sweet and bread eaten in secret is pleasant.
Proverbs 9:17

Have you ever had a secret stash of food?

Satan moves in the darkness. Sin comes about in secret. Food that no one sees us consume is okay. Calories don't count if it's eaten in secret, and yet that's the best tasting food in the world.

In the throes of an overeating compulsion, we hide candy in our desk at work. We keep muffins and candy at the back of our pantry at home praying that our mates don't find them.

One time, my oldest daughter found my stash of chocolate-covered cherries. Being a kind, considerate teenager, she washed them down the sink and into the garbage disposal. After all, she wanted to help me. I lost my temper because of a thoughtful gesture.

Our secret stashes save us when disappointment strikes or tragedy rocks our world. We turn to favorite foods.

What's the problem in that? We rely on candy and muffins when God wants us to trust Him instead. Secret food becomes our god.

Prayer: I trust in You, not food, to get me through the rough spots today.

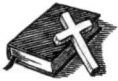

May 28

Secrets, Uncovered

So have no fear of them; for nothing is covered up that will not be uncovered, and nothing secret that will not become known. Matthew 10:26

A few years ago, I truly acted with insanity. Nearly every workday I stuffed into my mouth a bag of Reese's or a dozen donuts. Often, my husband traveled on his job. That gave me free license to sit in my chair and eat whatever I wanted. I went to bed at night miserable, not even able to sleep on my tummy as I preferred. Yet, even with feeling sick, I planned to run by the store on the way to work the next morning and pick up whatever sounded delicious to me at that moment.

Looking back, I sometimes wonder if I sought out jobs that left me alone for long periods of time. That wasn't a conscious thought, but perhaps the devil eased the way for me. When I had my favorite treat in my desk and a co-worker showed up unexpectedly, my ire flared. The compulsion affected my work, my relationships and, for sure, my ability to be a good wife and mother off the job.

When we overeat compulsively while alone, we feel safe from ridicule, but it doesn't keep off weight. Our body enlarges. Rolls of fat choke off our air and increase our blood pressure. Jesus warns us in the verse above. Sin will expose us. Secrets will be uncovered. Weight gain does reveal our overeating.

Prayer: Give me Your wisdom, Lord.

May 29

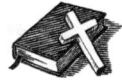

Reveal Your Secrets

For ye were sometimes darkness, but now are ye light in the Lord: walk as children of light. Ephesians 5:8

I hope you're not saying, "Oh, no, another day talking about secrets." If you are, perhaps, God is telling you that dishonesty is your problem.

Yesterday, we considered how God and natural rules of nature reveal our secret food addiction. The answer is revealing our own secrets. Truthfulness is the foundation for a walk with Christ.

The ABCs of salvation are:

A – Admit You're a Sinner

B – Believe Christ Died To Save You and Give You Eternal Life

C – Confess to Others That Christ Lives in Your Heart

The ABCs of healing from compulsive overeating are:

A – Admit the Problem Is More Than You Can Handle

B – Believe That God Can and Will Heal Your Compulsion

C – Confess to others our healing

To uncover our own secrets, we must start by overeating or eating the wrong things with someone watching. With me, it was my husband. The first time I ate a bag of candy in front of him, he said, "Guess you're off your diet today." Another time, he said, "That's not going to help you." Then, I prayed for God to give me courage, and God provided.

Sin brought into the open for all to see ceases to be as sweet and tempting. My husband quit making those comments, and my lapses decreased.

God knew the importance of bringing sin (overeating) into the light.

Prayer: Shine Your light on all I do, say or eat today.

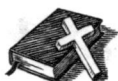

May 30

Freedom Tastes Better Than Sugar

If the Son therefore shall make you free, ye shall be free indeed.
John 8:36

My husband teases me that there is no such thing as too sweet for me.

My grandson once said, "I've never found a dessert I didn't like." I agree.

I love desserts—the sweeter, the better. For some of you, the salty taste of chips or crackers is what attracts you. Extreme flavors spark our taste buds—excess salty, sweet or spicy. However, phrasing goals in negative tones gets our hackles upturned.

Turn *this*:
> Stop eating sweets or limit sweets

into *this*
> Relish your newfound freedom and cherish your release from sugar addiction.

God provides true freedom from sin, addiction, and the devil's chains. Let me tell you, that's a wonderful feeling.

Prayer: Lord, I treasure freedom in You more than anything,
even the taste of my favorite foods.

May 31

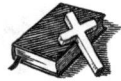

Are You a Plotter or Pantser?

Take therefore no thought for the morrow: for the morrow shall take thought for the things of itself. Sufficient unto the day is the evil thereof. Matthew 6:34

We who write use one of two methods. The first, writers call being a plotter. The other, we call being a pantser. I'm a plotter. When I start a new manuscript, I plan what will happen in each chapter and know how it will end. A friend of mine writes the first chapter by the "seat of her pants." She has a general idea of what the story is about, but has no idea how it will evolve or even how it will end.

Most of us go through our lives in one of these two methods. I plan everything; my day, my week, my year. I make lists, and I set goals.

Compulsive behavior bleeds over into other areas of life, but it ends up affecting our food. My compulsion to plan opens me up to frustration which then leads into compulsive overeating. Some overeaters struggle with compulsive shopping, gambling or another compulsive behavior. They lead from one to another.

Jesus warns us to not worry about tomorrow. Does that mean we should all be pantsers? Our total trust in God's ability to provide could lessen our need for incessant planning and our inability to handle detours. However, a true pantser might not plan enough to stay out of sand traps.

Prayer: Lord, help me rely so totally on You, today, that I might appear to not plan at all when, actually I make up suggested lists for the time ahead.

151

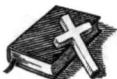

June 1

Capture That Thought

Finally, brethren, whatsoever things are true, whatsoever things are honest, whatsoever things are just, whatsoever things are pure, whatsoever things are lovely, whatsoever things are of good report; if there by any virtue, and if there be any praise, think on these things. Philippians 4:8

When we ask Jesus into our hearts, our spirits change immediately, but our minds change little by little for the rest of our lives. Selfishness can enter our minds. Satan can influence our thinking, depending on how wide we open the door.

Our minds are like the gates to our fort and become the battlefield for good versus evil. On no front is that more tangible than in the battle against compulsive overeating.

I've relapsed by dreaming of sitting alone, eating a whole bag of candy with no one seeing me. I've fallen by allowing anger to overwhelm me, causing me to fall prey to self pity.

Guard your gate, capture those defeating thoughts and think on healthy, worthwhile things. Only then can your healing remain steady. The enemy cannot enter the gate you defend with all your might.

Prayer: Today, remind me of the good in my life and help me avoid self pity and thoughts of overindulgence.

June 2

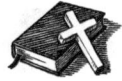

Take Your Vitamins

Through thy precepts, I get understanding; therefore I hate every false way. Thy word is a lamp unto my feet, and a light unto my path. Psalms 119:104,105

When we're pregnant or ill, the doctor asks if we're taking vitamins. Yet, most nutritionists advise taking a good multiple vitamin as a precaution even though we eat many fruits and vegetables that supply vitamins and minerals to our bodies. Our physical bodies require a certain amount of nutrients daily. Besides fruits and vegetables, we need grains for energy, proteins for building blocks and dairy for our bones.

Our spirits also need varied nutrients. We need wisdom and instruction, encouragement and advice, which are building materials for a strong Christian witness.

Addictive and compulsive personalities require more of this because of the hold our compulsion has on our spirits (mind). Like me, you perhaps have lived with food as your god for years. This strong hold is built-in and automatic, like a habit of destruction. When struggles threaten, we run to food unless the nourishment from God has become mightier.

- Take daily spiritual vitamins.
- Be prepared for rough spots.
- Let God be God in your life.

Prayer: Today, I study and soak up Your Word to use today, and whenever the need arises.

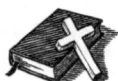

June 3

Raindrops On My Head

That ye may be the children of your Father which is in heaven; for he maketh his sun to rise on the evil, and on the good; and sendeth rain on the just and on the unjust. Matthew 5:45

In years past, the lyrics of a popular tune went, "Raindrops keep falling on my head, but that doesn't mean my eyes will soon be turning red." It goes on to say "Nothing's worrying me." I loved that song, made famous by B.J. Thomas.

Talking merely of a laid-back, take-life-as-it-comes type personality makes a nice idea but, in truth, severe troubles hit all of our lives. Without God, we're often unable to cope. Many turn to addictions. Some become bitter and harsh. The fact remains, as Jesus said above in Matthew, rain falls on everyone. The difference is whether Jesus walks through it with us or we deal with it by ourselves.

In past years, raindrops on my head sent me diving into a pan of fudge or a box of donuts. When I had become sated to the point of being stuffed, sedation stopped me. My mind condemned me. Anger boiled over at my actions. I forgot the real problem and lost all ability to pray and let God work on my behalf. Every thought and action focused on my fat and ugly body. I lost all benefit of God working through the rain to bring sunshine.

Prayer: Lord, the next time rain falls, I want You to take over, not my compulsion.

June 4

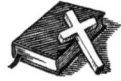

I'm Always Hungry

He satisfieth the longing soul, and filleth the hungry soul with goodness. Psalms 107:9

Sometimes, I really feel that I'm always hungry. When I've finished a big meal, a tasty treat still tempts me unless I feel sick. And believe me, I can eat until I'm sick.

An old saying goes, "A little food for thought gives some people indigestion." Unknown

When thoughts of rejection or loneliness roll through our minds, our stomachs somersault along with the mental gymnastics.

Thoughts on God and communing with Him applies antacid to our digestive system, thwarts our cravings, and calms the tumbling anxiety.

"Our lives are to be used and thus to be lived as fully as possible, and truly it seems that we are never so alive as when we concern ourselves with others." ~ *Henry Chapin*

God satisfies soul hunger.

Prayer: Lord, fill my soul hunger which stills my stomach needs.

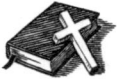

June 5

Human Failure

And the Lord, He it is that doth go before thee; He will be with thee, He will not fail thee, neither forsake thee; fear not, neither be dismayed. Deuteronomy 31:8

"Everyone cheats and lies," the man said. My husband and I looked at each other in disbelief. We didn't cheat or lie. What made the repairman think that? Needless to say, we decided against using him to fix our air conditioner. People judge others by their own experience. We assume everyone is like us.

A child raised by an abusive parent thinks his childhood is normal unless he spends time with other families. A woman expects all men to be like her man regardless of how cruel he is to her.

I feel I have the best husband in the world, but he's not without failure and fault. When I weighed two hundred and fifty, he grew impatient when I overate. He said things that hurt me. He regretted it and tried to do better, but he's human. Even now, when temptation teases my senses, he's not always there to snatch me out of harm's way. He's human.

Sometimes I feel as if I'm the biggest failure of all. I agree with Paul that "what I want to do, (always eat healthy and light) I don't do, and what I don't want to do, (stuff my face with sweets) sometimes, I do." What a relief to know that I rely on a God who never fails.

On earth, Jesus came across every type of temptation. He was hungry when Satan tempted Him to turn stones into bread, but He overcame temptation.

Victory in Jesus—that's not just a song, that's a promise. Thank You, Jesus.

Prayer: Help me follow the only perfect man.

June 6

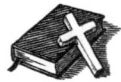

Diet is a Dirty Word

Beloved, I wish above all things that thou mayest prosper and be in health, even as thy soul prospereth. 3 John 1:2

Recently, a friend told me she'd decided to never diet again. "Diets bring out the rebellion in me. I end up eating worse than before the diet and gain even more weight."

I agree. I haven't dieted for eighteen years. Diet is a four letter word. Diets steal our joy and bring injury to our bodies and minds. God wants to bring healing to both.

> **D** – Deceit
> **I** – Internal Angst
> **E** – Envy
> **T** – Turmoil

Change this to freedom in Jesus—freedom to become whole.

> **H** – Healthy
> **E** – Energetic
> **A** – Alert
> **L** – Life

Quit dieting.

Ask the Lord what to eat. Find a way of eating that fits your lifestyle, not that of an actress or person selling a new potion.

Ask Jesus to show you a way of increasing activity. What do you like to do? Dance, tennis, golf, or just walk out with the birds singing?

Prayer: Lord, You created me as a unique individual. Be my eating and activity guide.

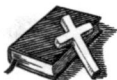

June 7

Perfectionism or Pride?

God opposes the proud, but gives grace to the humble.
1 Peter 5:6 NIV

I'm a perfectionist. Sometimes I think I'm not good at anything—being a mom, a wife, a friend, or even a Christian. I beat up myself. Yet, often, my problem stems from trying to do everything at once. I'm limited by human frailties. When I feel this way, am I experiencing humility or pride?

I fear that, in God's eyes, this form of self-denigration is pride, something God hates. The above verse states that God opposes the proud. I checked my thesaurus for a synonym for proud and found "arrogant, puffed-up, vainglorious, full of oneself."

Being a perfectionist means being full of ourselves. When we work hard to do a job "perfectly," we're puffed up and arrogant. When others don't do their jobs as well, we look down on them. When we don't do our jobs exactly right, we dislike ourselves. It's all about us. Is that not pride?

With humility, it's all about Jesus. We realize our limitations and don't run ourselves down because we understand we must rely on Christ.

The next time we describe ourselves as perfectionists, maybe we need to rethink that. Are we full of pride or humility? Reread the verse and remain humble.

Prayer: Lord, teach me humility whether I do well or not so well.

June 8

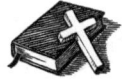

This Isn't a Day Trip

But the Lord is faithful, who shall stablish you, and keep you from evil. 2 Thessalonians 3:3

How many times have I gone on a diet to lose weight for a particular time or event? How often did I reach a low time and try the latest plan for losing? I looked at weight loss as a temporary period in my life. If I lost thirty pounds or sixty pounds, then my life would improve, and I could return to eating "normal."

I looked at a diet like I do a day trip.

An hour away from my home town is a national wild life refuge. There mountains, surrounded by plains, stretch for the sky, giving magnificent views. Buffaloes, longhorns and deer roam free. My husband and I take an occasional day trip there to enjoy God's wonderland. We leave home in the morning and hike while it's cool. We stop for lunch at a favorite landmark. We wade in the creek. We take pictures and visit the museum. In the afternoon, we return to our starting place and go back to normal.

With a journey of weight loss, we never return to normal. God's path to healing isn't a day trip but a lifetime journey. God establishes us day by day and keeps us from unhealthy practices until He takes us home to heaven.

Rid yourself of the notion of "going on a diet" and then stopping. We must never stop. Instead, we must turn and do a one, eighty life change.

Prayer: Lord, guide me every day of my life.

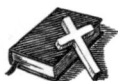

June 9

This is Hard Work

Come to me, all you who are weary and burdened, and I will give you rest. Take my yoke upon you and learn from me for I am gentle and humble in heart, and you will find rest for your soul. For my yoke is easy and my burden is light.
Matthew 11:28-30 NIV

Thomas Edison is quoted as saying "Opportunity is missed by most people because it comes dressed in overalls and looks like work."

That same thing can be said of weight loss. Following Christ to a healthy body is as simple as submitting to Him. But, it's not easy. It's no quick fix, no potion or single food or fact that solves the problem.

Losing weight with Christ involves the daily dedication of preparing your food in a proper fashion, praying every morning for the restraint of your runaway appetite, doing some form of activity to burn calories, and keeping an attitude of gratitude with no resentments regardless of what happens during your day.

- Hard work such as cooking a healthy meal instead of ordering pizza.
- Hard work such as choosing wisely in a restaurant instead of falling for the gimmick of one price for appetizer, entrée and dessert.
- Hard work such as taking a walk when you are tired and want to plop in your recliner.

Don your overalls, roll up your sleeves and put on your apron. Christ demands that we be serious before He intervenes to lighten our load.

Prayer: Lord, prepare my mind, take my sacrifice of praise, and lighten my load, today.

160

June 10

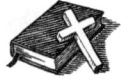

Act As If You've Got a Broken Wing

But unto you that fear my name shall the Sun of righteousness arise with healing in his wings; and ye shall go forth, and grow up as calves of the stall. Malachi 4:2

Across the parking lot waddled a mother duck with several ducklings following. We gathered outside to watch the spectacle. Holding herself at an odd angle, Mama Duck appeared to have a broken right wing. Our hearts reached out to this mother who, though hurt, still led her offspring to safety away from traffic.

When the troop of ducklings reached the side away from cars and nearest the lake, Mama Duck fluttered both wings in a wide arc covering her children. We laughed at the changing posture. Now that she had need of her wing to camouflage her ducklings, she demonstrated it was whole. With a seemingly broken wing while they trouped across the concrete, our focus was on her and kept our attention off the little ones. They remained safe.

God protects us, but we must "act as if" we have broken wings. While we do that, God does the work, heals the wound and accomplishes our goals.

Prayer: The world sees my broken wing today while You guide me to completeness.

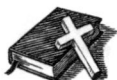

June 11

I Will Prevail

Nay, in all these things we are more than conquerors through Him that loved us. Romans 8:37

A reporter for our local TV news interviewed the fifth grade girl who had won the spelling bee contest. She would go on to Washington D.C. to compete.

"Were you scared?" the reporter asked.

The girl looked down. She shuffled her feet. "At first, I looked at the others around me so confident and thought I could never be any good. I wondered what I thought I was doing."

"After you spelled the third word correctly, I saw you stand straighter and face the questioner."

The young girl smiled, her dimples winking from each cheek. "Yes. At that point, I knew God was with me so I would prevail."

Sometimes, a loss of twenty, fifty or a hundred pounds sounds impossible. We might think, "What am I doing?" But, as we keep following Christ one step at a time, somewhere along the way, He'll make his presence real and impress our minds to the fact that "I will prevail."

We are conquerors because Jesus has already conquered it all.

Prayer: Today I will prevail with Jesus.

June 12

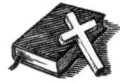

Stop Me now

And he said, My presence shall go with thee, and I will give thee rest. And he said unto him, If thy presence go not with me, carry us not up hence. Exodus 33:14,15

"It is not hard to live a Christian life; it is impossible." Anonymous

Like Moses—who traveled a hard, unknown path in the wilderness—I refuse to walk a single day without the Lord. Moses told God to stop him at the beginning unless He planned to go with him. God agreed to not only lead Moses, but give him rest along the way.

Today, I feel inadequate. Insufficient. Incapable. For many miles and multiple years, I have walked the path to weight loss. Still, whenever I don't "feel" God moving, I revert to a lack of confidence. Within myself, I would regain that ninety pounds in ninety days. Walking one more mile tires me, depletes my energy, leaving me with disbelief.

Daily, I pick up a picture taken at a shower for my firstborn grandbaby nineteen years ago. My engorged body in that picture reminds me of where I was. With each step, I travel an impossible road and faint with fatigue. I cry again, "Stop me now unless you lead."

Prayer: Today, I need Your rest and assurance.

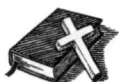

June 13

See No Evil, Hear No Evil, Speak No Evil

For he that will love life, and see good days, let him refrain his tongue from evil, and his lips that they speak no guile:
1 Peter 3:9

Many compulsive overeaters grew up in dysfunctional families. We moved into adulthood treating others the way our family treated us as children. We learned to build ourselves up by running others down. Belittling, venting anger, even telling lies interwove tentacles through our actions.

Even ones like me who had Christian parents who loved them learned love comes with judgment tied to its apron strings. I learned: *I love you, but I don't accept you.*

For years, I acted the part of the perfect Christian, but inside I had a deep, dark hole that fermented every good area of my life. Not only did I lie to others, I lied to myself. Holy Spirit conviction penetrated the lies and crushed my soul.

God showed me how to see no evil in others or myself.
God showed me how to hear no evil in others or myself.
God showed me how to speak no evil of others or myself.

My own lips should whisper blessing, not evil. How long has it been since you said to yourself, "I'm no good?"

Prayer: Help me speak no evil of myself, or others.

June 14

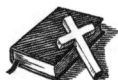

Let Me Off This Roller Coaster

Jesus Christ the same yesterday, and to day, and forever.
Hebrews 13:8

My emotional upheavals never stopped. From age eighteen to fifty, I bounced between the highs and lows. My roller coaster car never held at one level. At fifty, bad health challenged me to try again or suffer consequences, but I couldn't. Exhaustion and depression caused me to succumb.

I attended a Christian Weight Controllers class at my church. The teacher's words "Let go and let God" fueled my imagination.

During my struggles, I had prayed many times. I prayed to lose weight, I prayed for God to take away the craving for sweets, and I prayed for strength to follow a particular plan. Now, my words were different.

I looked to the ceiling and was honest. "Lord, I can't do it. If you don't change me from the inside out, I will die a lonely, overweight woman. It's up to You."

God took me up on my plea and showed Himself to be more powerful than I could describe. I've walked this journey with Him now for eighteen years. I lost ninety-five pounds and maintained it. Still, God didn't change my personality. He didn't yank me off the roller coaster. But just as I'm the same, Jesus is also the same.

I'm going through a low time mentally as I write this devotion. I wish my controlling instincts wouldn't overwhelm me, but they still do. God is prying my white knuckles from the control button. He desires that I feel the relief of submission once more. Are you there?

Prayer: Lord, I can't do it. Unless You take the controls, I'm
doomed. Help me be honest about that.

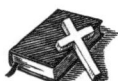

June 15

Safe From Winds

If a man abide not in me, he is cast forth as a branch, and is withered and men gather them and cast them into the fire, and they are burned. John 15:6

Memorial Day, 2011, my husband and I camped in our travel trailer. The winds were horrendous, the heat oppressive, in North Texas. Fires ravaged acres of land taking homes, barns, cattle, even some people in their paths.

Through the air sailed tumbleweeds and small limbs. On the west side of our trailer, I watched a small oak. The owners of the RV Park planted it for extra shade. When a gust of wind blasted from the south, a big cottonwood tree bowed over our patio and dropped cotton balls on our picnic table.

The oak, not more than four feet tall, braved the monster wind with strength and determination. The spindly branches folded but remained tight against the strength of a two-inch diameter trunk.

Though wind (or trials) buffeted that small tree, the branches remained in the trunk (or vine) and stayed firm, unmovable. God didn't promise I'd have no trials, no temptations, but He advised me to stay in Him to be able to withstand.

Forgoing daily quiet time with the Lord isn't an option for a compulsive person to prepare for the wind.

Prayer: I abide in You, today. It's the only way I stay safe when the winds blow.

June 16

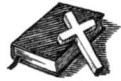

Do I Have to Admit it?

Admit your faults to one another and pray for each other so that you may be healed. The earnest prayer of a righteous man has great power and wonderful results. James 5:16 Recovery Bible

I remember one day locking the bathroom door and curling against the bathtub. My oldest daughter had softball practice, and the two younger ones were playing at the neighbor's house across the street. I was alone, just me and a box of chocolate-covered cherries and six Reese's peanut butter cups.

Even though my girls were away, they could at any time come bounding back in. I wanted to have time to destroy the evidence. I took with me two brown paper sacks and a book. I munched away devouring my problems one bite at a time. When my girls whooped as they entered the house, I stuffed the rest of the candy in one bag and hid it with the towels. The empty wrappers I put in the second sack, carried it as I walked out, and dropped it into the kitchen trash, all the time talking and listening while my daughters told their tales. I told no one my secret.

Step Five of Overeaters Anonymous says we confess our faults to ourselves, to God and to, at least, one other person.

Facing those shameful episodes ourselves is hard. A compulsive overeater lives in perpetual denial.

Then comes the time we must confess to God. Even though we know He forgives, we hate to put voice to our humiliation.

Ah, but telling another person—that's the hardest of all. But it's imperative. Only when we admit our faults and pray for each other do we release God's power into the circumstance.

Prayer: Remind me to live an open, honest life before God and man.

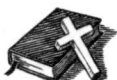

June 17

Do I Have to Love Her?

He that loveth not knoweth not God, for God is love. Beloved, if God so loved us, we ought also to love one another. 1 John 4:8,11

What about the boss that refuses to hire you because you're fat?

And the slim lady that makes catty references to how much you eat?

I think loving some people is impossible, just like controlling my food choices. Look at step number one of an anonymous program like Overeaters Anonymous:

- We admitted we were powerless over food; that our lives had become unmanageable.

Some personalities rankle and belittle. I could restate step one this way:

- I admit I was powerless over loving _____; that love for her/him had become impossible.

God is love. Through Christ, all things are possible. God can love that person through you and despite you if you let Him.

Since anger, resentment and envy can ruin any weight loss plan, we have three choices in which to handle unlovable people in our lives: a) we can avoid them; b) we can get mad and choke down food to get rid of our bad feelings; or c) we can let God love them through us. Since some are hard to avoid such as family or neighbors, that option rarely works. If we chose to quit eating ourselves into an early grave, option b is no good. Try option c and learn to love.

Prayer: Lord, I free You to love the ones in my life I can't love.

June 18

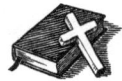

It's Time

For everything there is a season, and a time for every matter under heaven. Ecclesiastes 3:1

Nothing tastes as good as thin feels.

I learned this saying in Weight Watchers. It remains one of my favorites to remember and quote. A friend of mine changed it to say, "Nothing tastes as good as healthy feels."

King Solomon, the wisest man that ever lived, spoke the above words from life observation. My time for weight loss came at last. Maybe I took that long to learn to let God move in my life. Who knows? Can we hasten the season for us? I believe so.

Another saying I really like comes from Franklin F. Adams: *Health is the thing that makes you feel now is the best time of the year.*

When we improve our health, regardless of our season in life, a new world opens. Because we spend less time worrying about what we'll eat next, we have more time to create. Since we don't use as much time stopping for food and snacking, we expand our horizons. When my brain got off sugar, ideas popped like new adventures. Health makes any season the best time of all.

Could it be that this is your season for a new venture?

Prayer: Keep me off the sugar and fat and thereby free my mind to love whatever season is now.

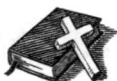

June 19

Patience, My Friend

For when the way is rough, your patience has a chance to grow. So let it grow, and don't try to squirm out of your problems. For when your patience is finally in full bloom, then, you will be ready for anything; strong in character; full and complete.
James 1:3,4 Recovery Bible

How many of us pray for patience?

How many of us do it the second time?

Like many early Christians, I prayed for patience and got trials. Why? Because that's what brings patience. But I hate trials.

Weight loss and changing habits require a lifetime. Setbacks and missteps dotted my pathway. Human nature drove me to my knees to pray "God, take away this craving," or "Lord, where were you when the temptation overpowered me?" God tells us to let the setbacks and stumbles come.

Last weekend presented one trial after another. My victories grew less each hour until I pulled out the frozen pizza Sunday night and ended the night with a bowl of oatmeal with tons of sugar. Hey, I couldn't find any other sweet in my house. In the past, I would face Monday morning with failure fatigue by going to the store to stock up on candy.

When I finished Sunday night's oatmeal, I prayed. "Lord, You've done it before. Teach me again. Clear my mind. Have Your will over the future choices I make."

Remember, always pray "God, take my life, my will, my choices." Every time I fail and ask God to lift me again, my faith blossoms, and my patience flourishes.

Patience is required. Prepare for patience. Expect trials.

Prayer: God take my life, my will, my choices today.

170

June 20

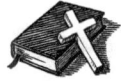

A Word about Bulimia and Anorexia

Thou blind Pharisee, cleanse first that which is within the cup and platter, that the outside of them may be clean also.
Matthew 23:26

Eating disorders come in one of three modes; anorexia, bulimia, and uncontrollable eating. I suffered the latter and put two hundred and fifty pounds on my five foot four inch frame.

Others have a stronger desire to look good on the outside even though the overeating compulsion drives them to more food. Bulimia (eating and taking laxatives to purge) and anorexia (eating and making yourself vomit) help some remain slim and svelte while overeating, but it can end in death.

For any of the eating disorders, our insides (resentments, envy, anger, putting food on the throne of our lives) look ugly, no matter how beautiful or fat our outsides.

Jesus told Pharisees and religious leaders during His earthly walk that was their problem. They wore religious robes and held prestige and respect among the people, but their insides pushed them away from the God they claimed to serve.

If you suffer from compulsive overeating (including bulimia and anorexia), Jesus asks you to look to Him. He's the great physician. Only He can heal and clean our insides.

Prayer: Look inside me today and keep me clean and beautiful before You.

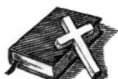

June 21

I Can't Do It

For by grace are ye saved through faith: and that not of your-
selves, It is the gift of God: Not of works, lest any man should
boast. Ephesians 2:8,9

I can do nothing to save myself. I can never summon enough
faith to give up something that has power over my mind. I am
captive to food. Thereby, I can't conquer the overeating compulsion. It is impossible.

THE ABOVE IS A FACTUAL STATEMENT.

Then, how, you might ask me, did I lose ninety-five pounds
and keep it off for eighteen years?

Here's an excerpt from one of my favorite books:

"We had been putting our final trust in our own faith, and
not in God's grace, and we had got the second things first."

From *Courage to Change,* by Bill Pittman and Dick B.

We can't. But God can.

Prayer: Without You, controlling food is impossible.

June 22

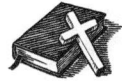

Jealousy

Don't envy evil men but continue to reverence the Lord at all time, for surely you have a wonderful future ahead of you. There is hope for you, yet! Proverbs 23:17,18 Life Recovery Bible

Skinny women make me sick. Correction: skinny women used to make me sick. When my food was out of control and my body not-so-pleasingly-plump, women who had no problem with food intimidated me. My struggles were insurmountable. To see my sister-in-law remain thin, though eating a candy bar every day, angered me.

When you're overweight and overwhelmed, the devil finds a foothold with envy. I could barely look at my daughter's mother-in-law because she was slim and petite. She pushed her food around the plate eating very little while I gulped huge portions until I was stuffed. Kindness oozed from this lady and her Christian witness strengthened many, yet I could only see that she looked good, and I hated her for it.

When the green-eyed monster of jealousy and envy pummels your mind, remember the verse above. I especially like the phrase, "There is hope for you, yet." The person you envy has other problems. Food is yours. Let the love of God flow and saturate your battered mind.

Let go, and let God love.

Let go, and let God choose.

Let go, and let God cleanse.

Let go.

Prayer: Lord, love through me today.

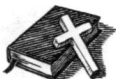

June 23

Fill Me Up

And blessed be his glorious name for ever; and let the whole earth be filled with his glory; Amen, and Amen. Psalms 72:19

Living in Texas heat, we feel blessed to have a swimming pool in our back yard. We built it fifteen years ago with a plastic liner. Hailed as a new design, it had no drain at the bottom. To empty it requires pumping out the water.

During these years, water left the pool through sloshing and evaporation. My husband added chemicals, measured them almost daily, and kept them in balance. All went well until this summer. The pool experts told us that certain chemicals had become so concentrated in our pool that nothing could purify the water and clean up our swimming area but pumping it out completely and filling it with new water.

While I watched that water pump out onto our lawn like liquid filth, I thought of all the years of putting in stuff that clouded and made toxic our pool. When it finished, we poured fresh water into the liner. The pool was filled with the newness of clean water.

Isn't that like our lives? We drift along for years, pouring more and more "junk" into ourselves. We reach the point where it's so concentrated that it brings destruction and contamination. We empty out the bad stuff, and God pours in His newness of spirit.

Years of compulsive overeating requires us to clear our bodies of sugars and fats, our minds of filthy thinking, and our spirits of addiction.

Prayer: Lord, help me pump out the old so that You may pour in the new.

June 24

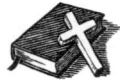

How long?

This is the day the Lord hath made; let us rejoice and be glad in it. Psalms 118:24.

In the field of psychology, it is well known that the weight of the burden isn't nearly as important as how long we've carried the load. A counselor first explores your childhood because burdens carried that many years cause the most stress or can be the underlying cause of great difficulties.

Compulsive overeaters eat over stress, whether it's because we had a bad day at work or because we argued with our mates ten years ago. The ten-year stressor induces more overeating, but the bad day can trigger the deeply-buried stress already in our lives.

Many compulsive overeaters require one-on-one counseling. Stress brought about from dysfunctional childhood homes drives many to stuff their feelings with a heaping spoonful of dessert. If we are to heal, we must uncover the source of our stress. Once we do that and lay it before the Lord, we must rely each day thereafter on God's joy.

Wake up each morning with the verse above on your lips. It will transform your life. Trust God's joy and His peace to ferret out remaining stress and provide a source to handle the day-by-day bad days.

Prayer: Thank You, Lord, for my emotional healing now and every day.

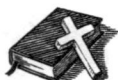

June 25

Dance More

Let them praise his name with dancing, and make music to him with tambourine and harp. Psalms 149:3 NIV

My parents raised me in a church which preached that dancing was wrong. But the devil takes mere food, the sustenance of life, and uses it for evil.

We bless our food. We give glory to God for healthy, colorful, good tasting morsels. We thank God for meals that delight the sense of taste and smell.

We dance before the Lord to give Him praise, but we can also use dance to move our bodies in exercise. Recently, at our church, we had a Zumbathon® as a youth fundraiser. I thanked the lady who planned something that helped us physically instead of doing harm. How many times do church groups sell cakes, or plan a meal to raise money or have fellowship? These activities can give pleasure but can also bring affliction, depression, and give the devil a stronghold. Dancing for fun and exercise can help us or hurt us. But why place it in the hurt column without ever giving it a chance?

Recently a country western song compared dancing with enjoying life. The lyrics referenced praying that you dance.

Looking for a new activity to help your weight loss, your emotional outlook and a chance for sheer enjoyment? Join a Zumba® class, learn to line dance, go to the Y for aerobics, or just dance around your house as you clean.

You might also pray, praise, and dance before the Lord.

Prayer: Thank you, Lord, that dance can be helpful.

June 26

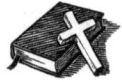

Unshakeable Faith

(For we walk by faith, not by sight). 2 Corinthians 5:7

Recently, I read in one of my favorite books, *Courage to Change,* "The real enemy of faith is not reason, but inexperience." I've read those words often, but they never cease to stop and make me think.

Scientists work on a hypothesis and seek to either prove or disprove a theory. When a science major studies, he listens to his professor and follows through with the guidelines suggested. In most cases, the student proves the professor knows what he's talking about. Why? Because the professor has tried it.

To reach the point of faith without sight, we first listen to a teacher or preacher or saint about God's answer to their prayers. Then, we follow their guidelines and what happens? God answers our prayers. We learn from experience.

People perish for lack of experience. Try trusting Him. Prove or disprove He's faithful with your money, your food, your family, your life. The more times you experience God's faithfulness, the more unshakeable your faith becomes, regardless of bad things happening.

Prayer: Lord, I don't know how You can stop me from overeating today, but You've got to do it. I can't.

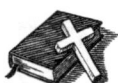

June 27

Maybe I Should Strive to Be Fat

And the Lord shall guide thee continually, and satisfy thy soul in drought, and make fat thy bones; and thou shall be like a watered garden and like a spring of water whose waters fail not. Isaiah 58:11

This verse spoke to me today. Maybe I've been looking at my problem upside-down. Instead of thinking I want to be thin, I'll strive to be fat.

In the Bible, fatness translates to healthiness, strength, vigor, prosperity, while thinness equates to weakness, fragility, unhealthy living, and poverty.

If we follow the Lord *CONTINUALLY*, He will make us fat. He will chase away the drought through Holy Spirit fire, spiritual renewal, and refreshing.

In Fort Worth, the botanical gardens include many ponds, waterfalls and fountains. Even on hot days, a cool mist sprinkles our bodies and calms our minds. We have friends that added several fish ponds to their back yard garden. This addition keeps their plants watered and brings contentment from sitting in their garden.

The word picture of this verse is beautiful. Meditate on it today. Seek for God's "fatness of the bones."

Prayer: As I follow You, make me fat and contented in You.

June 28

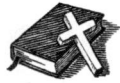

I Win

No weapon forged against you will prevail. Isaiah 54:17

In Satan's arsenal many weapons reside, ready to do damage. Though he doesn't have all knowledge like God, he possesses much insight into the minds of men. For me, temptation comes in the form of food, or worry, or angry outbursts. The devil brings a weapon against me when I'm the most weak or vulnerable.

The above verse is one I can quote and rely on at that time. Memorizing Scripture holds us steady. This verse is short and to the point. With God, success comes—no matter what.

A friend of mine loves to say "I've read the back of the Bible, and we win."

Jesus faced temptation on earth so that He would understand what we go through. He is our example. Look at how he faced temptation in the wilderness. He quoted Scripture.

Next time the devil pulls out the weapon of candy to give you energy when you're tired, or anger when a fellow Christian tramples your good name, quote that Scripture. Prayers are more powerful when we proclaim God's word. Our children use our words against us when we try to correct or teach them. Do the same with God.

The next time you face temptation, ask God to save you because "You promised no weapon would prevail against me." Power up your prayers with the Word.

Prayer: Keep me safe from temptation.

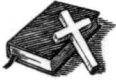

June 29

My Stuff is Holding me Back

And David said unto his men, Gird ye on every man his sword. And they girded on every man his sword; and David also girded on his sword; and there went up after David about four hundred men and two hundred abode by the stuff. 1 Samuel 25:13

Stuff? Stuff held back a third of David's troops from fighting that day. Let me read that again. David put on his sword to fight the enemy and led two-thirds of his men into war. Clearly, he could not use some of his men because of stuff.

Last Sunday, my pastor preached on "What stuff holds you back?" That thought resonated with me because, even now after I've retired from my day job, I have to do a priority list at least once a year. I write down everything I do on a regular basis. My life choices range from quiet time with the Lord to traveling, reading for pleasure, group meetings, housecleaning, visiting grown children, line dancing, Bible study, prayer meeting, talking with hubby and Facebook, along with too many more items to count. Then, I number my list. First is quiet time with God, then talking with hubby, etc.

We require a priority list because our stuff jams our lives too full. What does that have to do with being an overeater? Why must we tabulate our choices?

Because:

1. We tend to overeat when we're overwhelmed.
2. We spend too much time on the inconsequential and not enough on the most important, then we get depressed.
3. We hate to say no to something good, so we must prepare for that moment when we're asked. We must visualize action.
4. We desire to be utilized for God to our fullest capabilities. (Not at two-thirds of potential.)

Prayer: Control my stuff and use me to my fullest.

180

June 30

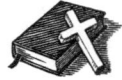

Driven by Reckless Lust

They don't care anymore about right and wrong and have given themselves over to impure ways. They stop at nothing, being driven by their evil minds and reckless lusts.
Ephesians 4:19 Life Recovery Bible

As a child, I gave my heart to Christ. During college, I drifted away but then rededicated my life to Him. The last thing I expected to be accused of was lust.

Webster's New World Dictionary defines lust as: 1) bodily appetite or 2) overwhelming desire. *Roget's Super Thesaurus* gives several synonyms including hunger, urge, craving.

Craving? Now we're talking something every compulsive overeater understands. Is that not the definition? I crave certain foods with an overwhelming desire or appetite until I get it and binge or eat without control. If that's not reckless lust, what's a better comparison?

In His Word, God gave the example of Eve in Genesis 3:6. Eve lusted after that forbidden fruit because she saw that it was good for food, and pleasant to the eye, and would make her wise. With me, a donut oozes cream filling, making it pleasant to look at, good to eat and it would calm my stress. I lust for the donut.

Are you driven by your reckless lusts?

Prayer: Lord, deliver me from lust and instead fill me with Your joy.

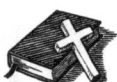

July 1

Let God Hold the Steering Wheel

For as the heavens are higher than the earth, so are my ways higher than your ways, and my thoughts than your thoughts.
Isaiah 55:9

When my addiction tangled me in its throes, psychologists told me I needed to think positively. Sermons convicted me of my pride and obsessions. My husband couldn't understand why I would stuff myself with food when I always got sick after-ward. My thoughts were flawed, but I couldn't change how I felt.

We fight compulsive overeating on two fronts; huge appe-tite and emotional imbalance. Emotions drive us to believe we can overcome the appetite but, at the same time, uncontrol-lable emotions fuel our appetites.

"You may not have joy at the moment. Your soul may not be flooded with peace. In fact, you may still have turmoil in your soul. If that is the case, stay rooted firmly in his Word. Stop trying to think your way through it." David Wilkerson, the founder of Teen Challenge.

Stop trying to think your way through your compulsion to overeat. Stop looking for a new diet, a good exercise class or even thinking positively about overcoming the imbalance of your emotional flood.

Stay in the Word. Let it fill your mind.

Give God the wheel. Lean back and enjoy the ride.

Your thinking, whether good or bad, will never succeed because you don't think like God.

Prayer: Take the wheel of my life. I made a mess of driving.

182

July 2

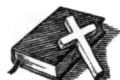

I've Failed

He that diggeth a pit shall fall into it; and whoso breaketh an hedge, a serpent shall bite him. Ecclesiastes 10:8

Not doing what we know we must do to refrain from compulsive overeating = digging a pit.

Skipping several days without waiting on God = breaking up the hedge He put around us.

True confession time:

Yesterday, I completed five days with grandkids and did no writing, no reading, and no quiet time with God. That doesn't work for me. I must have time away with God every day.

The ironic thing is that I can keep under God's protection and strength for awhile and don't realize I'm growing weaker. All the time I camped and played with the kids, I ate healthy and light and, of course, got plenty of activity.

Still, weakness crept into my mind, sneaky as in all of Satan's devices. I've been going on the steam power gleaned a few days ago, oblivious that it's nearly expired—not unlike taking medicine that heals me while being blinded that it's the last pill.

Answer to failure:

Stop where you are. Remedy what you're ruining. Go to Jesus NOW.

The best lesson I've learned is I can change course on Saturday and not wait until Monday, or 4 p.m. and not wait until the next day. DO IT NOW.

Prayer: Lord, thank you for once again giving me a reminder of why I need You, and picking me up from the ditch immediately.

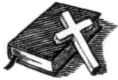

July 3

Walk in the Spirit

For they that are after the flesh do mind the things of the flesh; but they that are after the Spirit the things of the Spirit.
Romans 8:5

List ten things in life most important to you. Now look at your list. The expression "What would Jesus do?" has been over-used but is still worth thinking about. How many items on your list would Jesus count as valuable?

How do you spend your time? your money? your thoughts?

Be honest. Is food on your list? I would have to say it still makes my top ten. I find myself often thinking what to eat, what to cook, where to go out to eat or actually eating or snacking. When I was in trouble or sad, or down about something, food used to be my first thought. I'm far from perfect in this category, but now my first focus is to run to God and beg for help.

The biggest difference for a compulsive overeater before recovery and in recovery is where you turn when you want to eat everything in sight.

It's not who runs your eating, it's who you run to with your eating.

Stay in the Spirit. The flesh is weak.

Prayer: Lord, thanks for opening Your arms when I run to You.

July 4

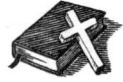

Remove My Chains

For I see that you are full of bitterness and captive to sin.
Acts 8:23 NIV

When we're tied in knots because of compulsive overeating, we are captive to Satan's seductive tactics.

Cranky
Harmful
Anxious
Ire
No Energy
Suicidal

Bottom
Overwhelmed
Useless
Narcissistic
Despairing

I love the words that go along with the song "Amazing Grace" presented by Chris Tomlin:

My chains are gone.
I've been set free.
My God, My Savior
Has rescued Me.
And like a flood
His mercy reigns.
Unending love,
Amazing Grace.

Prayer: Lord, thank You for Your mercy every day.

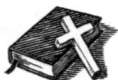

July 5

Stay Free

Stand fast therefore in the liberty wherewith Christ hath made us free, and be not entangled again with the yoke of bondage.
Galatians 5:1

FREEDOM A sermon presented by a guest preacher this morning was on freedom. He told the story of how "The Star-Spangled Banner" song came into being. It's a fascinating story if you haven't read it lately. The beginning and preservation of the United States of America is all about freedom—we wanted freedom to worship, to excel, to govern ourselves.

As individuals, we desire freedom above all things. Many think that means doing whatever we want. The true meaning of freedom is only recognized through doing the will of God. When I ate whatever I wanted to eat, the food enslaved me. I lost my freedom. Freedom in Jesus may seem in the beginning giving up what we want (i.e. donuts, Reese's candy), but only through giving up what we think we want can we receive what we need.

FREEDOM RELEASE

F ull life	**R** est
R elationship with Christ	**E** nergy
E steem	**L** ife
E ternity	**E** verything
D esire of the heart	**A** we of God
O ut of chains	**S** ubmission
M atter	**E** nthusiasm

Prayer: Thank You, Lord, for the easy yoke You supply.

July 6

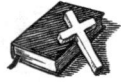

Let Me Be Willing.

Restore to me the joy of your salvation, and grant me a willing spirit to sustain me. Psalms 51:12 NIV

All good and proper gifts come from heaven. Jesus tells us we must have faith to please God but then reminds us that even our faith comes from God.

God saved me while I was yet in sin. Thanks be to Him, I didn't have to clean up my life before He would save me. No, He retrieved me from the trash heap, with the stink of garbage still clinging to my thoughts, saved me, and offered to help me with my struggles.

To follow God, even in taking food out of God's place, we require a willing spirit—willing to follow Christ' lead. Yet when we truly release our wills to God, He provides even the continued willing spirit.

When we grow weary of not eating as much as we want, when the scale mocks our attempts, or when we long to quit, God restores our joy. We long for a permanent, once-and-for-all remedy, but God wants our day-to-day dependence. When the Israelites crossed the desert, God supplied food, clothing and protection for the entire trip—but not in one lump blessing. Like them, He desires we ask Him daily for what only He can give.

We yield to the day-to-day walk only after reaching the bottom and realizing God alone can provide our joy, our hope and our willingness.

Prayer: Grant me a willing heart.

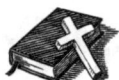

July 7

Never Too Bad

Come, let's talk this over! Says the Lord; no matter how deep the stain of your sins, I can take it out and make you as clean as freshly fallen snow. Even if you are stained as red as crimson, I can make you white as wool. Isaiah 1:18 Life Recovery Bible

What a promise! I love all of God's promises, but if I had to stand on just one, that would be it.

Are you a murderer? Have you tortured and killed? What about theft—how much have you stolen? No? Ah, but have you lied? Have you denigrated God's creation? Have you built up resentment or bitterness in your heart? Have you envied fellow Christians or coveted their recognition?

When we first ask God to help us, we know we're through, beaten-up, and useless. If we keep working at this diet thing, we would be over five hundred pounds by old age. Some of us wanted to kill ourselves.

My life totaled fifty years of dieting, binging, and dieting again. My poor body wouldn't release one pound more, no matter what I ate. Though I begged God to help me, the heavens remained silent. I was like the child who asked her father to fix her toy but wouldn't let go of it for him to start.

I entered the room for a first Christian Weight Controller class at our church because I didn't know what else to do. I realized I could no longer live the way I was going. I had no answer. I attended because my friends did. Why not? I could again claim I'd tried, but I knew it wouldn't help.

One night, God met me with that Scripture challenge. Nothing in my life was too hard for God to fix. God could and would clean every sin. And He did.

Prayer: Clean me daily.

July 8

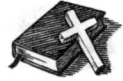

One Moment at a Time

In all thy ways acknowledge him, and he shall direct thy paths.
Proverbs 3:6

At the beginning of January, eighteen years ago, I joined a Christian Weight Controllers class. I held no enthusiasm and very little hope. I sought camaraderie with other compulsive overeaters, I went through the motions of excitement, but I felt beat, defeated, at bottom.

On the first day, I told God, "I'll eat this for breakfast, but after that, I'm eating what I want. If you can change me, do so. I can't." Mid-morning came. I told God, "I'll eat another fruit, but I'm having pizza for lunch because I'm not willing to give it up unless you change me." By lunchtime, a friend called me to meet her at the mall to walk. I refused because it wouldn't leave me enough time to eat lunch, but it got me thinking about walking. I don't remember what I had to eat, but it wasn't pizza.

When the next day started, I realized I had eaten according to the American Diabetic exchange diet plan for one whole day without planning on it. I packed a lunch and called my friend for a walking lunch date.

The day after, I planned on a stopover at my favorite donut shop on the way to work. When I drove into the parking lot at work, I realized I forgot to stop for my treat.

By this time, I began to wonder. Is that daily turning it over to God really working?

The above paragraphs are a simplified version of my weight loss journey, but they give an example of how I let go and let God, and He faithfully "directed my path." I didn't do anything but blindly follow.

Prayer: I am weak and powerless. Continue to guide me, Lord.

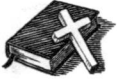

July 9

Unrelenting will

I thank God through Jesus Christ, our Lord: So then with the mind I myself serve the law of God; but with the flesh: the law of sin. Romans 7:18

Our minds literally set in motion whatever we unrelentingly will to happen, whether good or bad. Our flesh desires feelings and food contrary to God's will, but if we indulge in them, they end in sin. When we deliberately aim to do God's will, the result succeeds and serves God.

"We are more than our environment . . . a dream, backed by an unrelenting will to attain it, is truly a reality within imminent arrival." Anonymous

One of my favorite motivational books is *Psycho-Cybernetics* by Maxwell Maltz. It isn't a Christian book, but the principles he teach can be applied to committing your life and will to God. Maltz describes "victory through surrender" in this manner: "Give up the feeling of responsibility, let go your hold, resign the care of your destiny to higher power, be genuinely indifferent as to what becomes of it all."

The Bible gave us the remedy for an unrelenting will bent on overeating: "Be still and know God." We use the term, "let go and let God."

Prayer: I ask help to surrender daily to Your will, not mine.

July 10

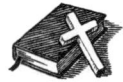

Oleanders and Weight Loss

*...Why be discouraged and sad? Hope in God! I shall yet praise
him again. Yes, I shall again praise him for his help.*
Psalms 42:4 Life Recovery Bible

God amazes and encourages us. In the midst of trials and
turmoil, God sends small reminders that He knows our plight
and feels our pain.

One summer vacation, our sprinkler system failed and our
lawn went waterless. My husband grieved. He watered deeply
and often, but the brown grass and trees prematurely losing
their leaves mocked his every effort. We prayed for our yard.
Remember, God cares about the little things that trouble us.

Two days later, an oleander bush broke into profuse
blooms. It was like a rainbow after the storm for my husband.
God encouraged him. We knew God cared.

In the beginning we may lose weight every week. Over time
the loss slows. Sometimes we gain. Many times we fall from the
boat and then God sends a raft.

Once despondency nagged my mind more than usual. I ate
well for six weeks with no loss. Then, I prayed. "I can't change
anything about my body. I'm a weak vessel tossed by frustration. Search my mind for evidence of resentment or envy.
Examine my body for lack of sleep or proper nourishment. Heal
the anger welling in my mind."

God's silence was deafening. I set out a fleece.

"I need to see a dip in the scale tomorrow to let me know
You're there." The next day I dropped four pounds.

A lady in our church is known for one particular song. Many
times, we request "He'll do it again."

*Prayer: We need Your encouragement today and again
tomorrow.*

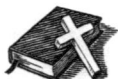

July 11

Start Again

Therefore we are buried with him by baptism unto death: that like as Christ was raised up from the dead by the glory of the Father, even so we also should walk in newness of life.
Romans 6:4

Sometimes we must start again.

We may turn our eating to God and follow His guidance for months or years but then cares of life or emotions set on edge puts us wandering the woods. As a lost boy scout who searches for his troop, we wear ourselves out seeking peace.

At times like that, we must start at the beginning. When we go to clean out a closet, these are the steps we take:

1. Pull everything out to see what's there.
2. Place stuff in three piles and make decisions on:
   - Things to throw away.
   - Things to give to someone else.
   - Things to put back in the closet.
3. Add new things.

When we start again from feeling overwhelmed and/or overeating, we use the same three steps:

1. List everything you do and every concern you have.
2. Prioritize everything taking up space in your life or your mind and classify in three ways.
   - Rid yourself of bad emotions by asking God's help and eliminate some jobs with God's guidance.
   - Delegate jobs where you can.
   - Recommit to the God-directed items remaining.
3. Add joy and peace that God wants to give you.

Prayer: Lord, guide me to newness in my walk.

July 12

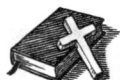

Fortify the Fortress around Me

He shall call upon me; and I will answer him; I will be with him in trouble; I will deliver him and honor him. Psalms 91:15

God promises to fight and defeat every enemy that comes against us. But, only if we ask Him.

My husband and I cruised the Caribbean on a ship going to Puerto Rico. We took a walking tour of downtown old San Juan. On a point overlooking the ocean, tourists visit El Morro, at one time a formidable defensive fortress for the island. Spanish inhabitants built this fort in 1589. History tells us it withstood many assaults, but once in 1598, even this fort was defeated in an overland attack.

God's fortress stands through EVERY attack the enemy can assail. No human or anything devised of men can hold up. But, God will not go against our will. Like a gentleman, He waits for an invitation.

An anonymous quote that I like is humorous but meaningful:

"When one reaches the so-called 'jumping-off point,' he discovers that by God's gracious goodness ... the world is round."

Take a chance on God. He always protects.

Prayer: I pray to rely on Your defense today.

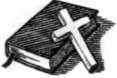

July 13

It's Delicious

Thou preparest a table before me in the presence of mine enemies; thou anointest my head with oil; my cup runneth over.
Psalms 23:5

Parties, fellowships, and pot-lucks can try our determination faster than anything—and our churches abound with such.

The National Health and Nutrition Survey in 2004 told us 133.6 million (66%) adult Americans were obese or overweight. A Purdue University study indicates conservative churches such as Southern Baptist, Assembly of God, and Church of God fight this battle more often. Richard Kreider of Baylor University gives further insight into this. These denominations "avoid dancing, tobacco and alcohol, but give no guidelines for over-eating." He goes on to say our churches more often attract with food, not action events.

Church functions served as an enemy to me for years. Any woman worth her salt prepared the best tasting dish she had for these events. And I felt duty-bound to try them all. Like the Baylor survey suggests, my righteousness included no smoking, no drinking, and a long list of "nos," but eating was okay.

But **GOD** serves His delicious food to **Me** in the presence of others who overeat or tease me (my enemies).

Prayer: Praise Your name for delicious, healthy foods.

July 14

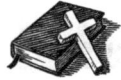

I Can't Go On

Each time he said "No, but I am with you; that is all you need, my
power shows up best in weak people."
2 Corinthians 12:9 Life Recovery Bible

I volunteer to be that weak person. How about you?

In prior verses, the apostle Paul begs God to rid him of a thorn in his flesh, but God refuses. In this verse though, God promises to be with him. For years, I begged God to eliminate my compulsive personality, to take away my craving for sweets, but God said "No."

Now, through my years since God's healing, I still reach points where I feel I can no longer go on. Why do I have to limit my portions while others eat all they want? It's not fair. I want to eat all the things I like. And I don't want to exercise today.

I give up. God convicts me of the old resentments and envy accumulating. He takes me back to that verse in Corinthians. When I'm at my weakest, God can be strong in me if I let Him.

Go back to the beginning. Turn your will, your life, and your choices to His care, and watch Him work miracles.

Sometimes, God says "No," so He can demonstrate His glory in us.

Prayer: Lord, be strong through me today.

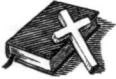

July 15

What Makes Me Think
This Will Continue?

Being confident of this very thing, that he which hath begun a good work in you will perform it until the day of Jesus Christ.
Philippians 1:6

Only twenty per cent of people who lose weight will keep it off. Many join a clinic and become svelte, but then pounds stack up again. Their demeanor loses its luster. Their shoulders slump. They remain in the background.

When I see this, I think of the old adage, "There by the grace of God, go I." This is more than a cliché. This is my life's truth.

Eighteen years ago, when the needle on the scale dropped again and again, belief in lasting help eluded me. I had followed that road too many times. January passed again. I celebrated my first anniversary since joining the Christian weight loss group. I had dropped forty-eight pounds and teetered close to the two hundred mark on the scale. Excitement spurred me to further accomplishments. I hadn't weighed below two hundred in twenty years. Was it possible?

I neared that mark and gained again, following this pattern for several weeks. But, the time came that I crossed that threshold. The scale showed 198 ½. By this time, our leader had moved and I was teaching the class. I began to believe.

What was the difference this time?

My confidence held on to God. I'd already proven I couldn't do it. When God starts a work, He is able to continue it. Our part is to hold onto Him with all our might.

Prayer: Lord, hold to me as I hold to You.

July 16

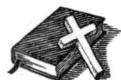

Watch the Stripes

*I will instruct thee and teach thee in the way which thou shalt go;
I will guide thee with mine eye. Psalms 32:8*

In my haste to be all things to all people, my life often veers too far to one side or the other. Highway departments paint a center stripe on narrow roads and several stripes on freeways. Without these, one car might swerve into another. Center stripes help stop head-on collisions. The darker the night, the more we need stripes with reflective paint or pegs. Have you ever thought about who decided to paint stripes on highways? When did that become necessary?

In the early 1900s, our roads consisted mostly of dirt or sand. Traffic meant horses or carriages. Interestingly enough, bicyclers first brought attention to the need for better roads in 1897. With the invention of the Model T, the US government realized a need for standardization of the road system. A simple idea like stripes on the highways minimizes collisions and gives guidance on your travels.

God's word and instruction in prayer is a Christian's stripe on the pathway of life. We tend to get too far in one direction, compensate, and then go too far in the other. Twelve-step programs use the mantra, "First Things First" to remind us to take care of our recovery first, then all things will fall in place. God tells us to "Seek first the kingdom of God."

Focus on God (the stripe). He will tell you when your compass is off base. Then, you can adjust and stay on the right road. Your spiritual recovery must always be your first focus.

Prayer: Help me keep first things first today.

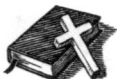

July 17

On Eagle's Wings

Ye have seen what I did unto the Egyptians; and how I bare you on eagles' wings, and brought you unto myself. Exodus 19:4

On a recent trip to the Rocky Mountains of Colorado, my husband and I watched the golden eagles. Vallecito Lake area, near Durango, experienced the Missionary Ridge fire in 2002 that gutted much of their forest. Tall, leafless trees left by the fire provide places that the eagles build nests. We spotted two, one with baby eagles in it and the mama and papa flying in and out with food.

We loved driving by the trees and watching for the birds to swoop to the nest. Eagles prefer high, secluded spots. When the time comes for their babies to fly, mama eagle pushes them from the nest. She watches carefully. If the young bird drops too fast, she sweeps under the baby, balances it on her wings, and flies back to the beginning. Then, they start the process over again.

God pushes us into the world but remains ever watchful. When we falter, He carries us up as on eagles' wings to safe ground. Then, we start again.

I love this picture. I am never alone. I can look to Him for deliverance at any point. If I do, He will not allow me to drop.

Prayer: I take hope when I spot an eagle that You created.

July 18

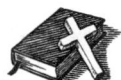

True Trust

Trust in the Lord with all thine heart, and lean not unto thine own understanding. Proverbs 3:5

When our three girls were young, we vacationed every summer. The mountains beckoned us—with beautiful scenery for Charles and I, horseback riding for the oldest girl, and kid activities for the two youngest. Sometimes we drove a jeep or rented a bicycle, but most often we hiked. I'm afraid of heights, so my husband often scared me.

He ventured up and down rocks, to the very precipice, edging to a narrow ledge, or crossing a rope bridge over a deep canyon. Our two oldest girls followed every spot his foot took in front of them. They seemed to believe that if they stepped exactly as he did, they would remain safe. The younger girl's feet once slipped, but Charles caught her and carried her back to me.

The poem of "Footprints of Christ" ministers to many. If we could view the sands of our timeline, sometimes we'd see only one set of footprints because, during that time, Jesus carried us.

If we keep our eyes on the steps of Jesus and walk as he does we will not falter. Think of that picture when you're having a bad day and want to eat everything imaginable. Look at Jesus. Where is His next foothold in the rocks? If we're following when the incline worsens, He will carry us to keep us safe.

Prayer: Help me watch Your steps and follow closely behind You.

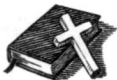

July 19

Big Mouth and Busybodies

To the shelter of your presence you hide them from the intrigues of men; in your dwelling you keep them safe from accusing tongues. Psalms 31:20

Hateful, malicious words hurt our feelings and destroy our hope. Even when we eat well and exercise, no one can lose weight all at once. Our self-esteem nosedives. Anger builds. We seek to soothe our emotions with more food.

Big mouths and busybodies have no place in church. Yet, that's where we often encounter them. To succeed, we must rise above the petty prejudice, understanding it for what it is— a poor attempt to build their own self worth.

God shelters us from the mean spirits and unkind remarks. Only He can renew our hope when it's thrown to the ground and trampled.

God's Word tops everything as a resource for guidance, but other books help. I recommend an in-depth journal encounter titled *Locked Up for Eating Too Much: The Diary of a Food Addict in Rehab* by Debbie Danowski, Ph.D.

Like me, some of you might identify with Dr. Danowski.

Prayer: Shelter me from cruel tongues.

July 20

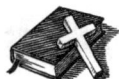

100%

And he said unto his disciples, 'Therefore, I say unto you, take no thought for your life; what ye shall eat; neither for the body, what ye shall put on. Luke 12:22

God wishes to be our all. He wants 100% of our honor, our worship. Jesus tells us to not worry about our food or our clothes. He goes on to remind us to look to Him. God supplies everything we need.

100% – All – Everything

"God wants it all. But, when we make Him the master of our minds, we are free from the pull of food. Sounds good to me! Since we are going to be a slave to one or the other, I choose God." *The Weigh Down Diet by* Gwen Shamblin

Like Ms. Shamblin says in her book, the more we dwell on God, the stronger the pull or drive to draw closer. But the more we think on a food that we like, the stronger the desire becomes for that food. Gradually, those cravings drive a wedge between us and God's best.

How much of this problem does He want us to give to Him?

Prayer: Lord, I look to You for everything.

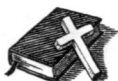

July 21

Three Steps to Victory

Submit yourselves therefore to God. Resist the devil, and he will flee from you. Draw nigh to God, and he will draw nigh to you . . . .
James 4:7,8a

Grow a good marriage with communication. Without knowing the heart of your mate, you are sure to often displease him or her. Any relationship gains strength by spending time together and talking about all the things that matter to you.

My husband and I use a clichéd saying for my daughter and granddaughter. "They're like mixing oil and water." This is our way of saying they storm into each other with heightened anger, tongue-lashings and misunderstandings. They keep secret much of their lives, and this causes the other one not to grasp the motive or reality of what's happening.

To expect God to help us when the devil attacks, we must remain close and communicate to follow His leading. Note the above verse holds three steps:

1. Resist the devil—Flee, use the Scripture to battle, don't put yourself into difficult situations.
2. Submit to God—Allow Him to direct you even when your flesh is defiant; yield as you would to oncoming traffic.
3. Draw close to God—Before the devil strikes, keep the relationship and communication lines open.

This is God's three-step plan to remaining victorious over the devil's snare of food worship in your life.

Prayer: Let's talk, Lord.

July 22

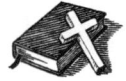

De-stress

Casting all your care upon Him; for careth for you. 1 Peter 5:7

Stress complicates any weight loss plan.

Here's the prescription to **DE-STRESS:**

> **D**ependence on God
> **E**verything (He is).
> **S**implify
> **T**ime spent with God
> **R**ead God's Word
> **E**liminate non-priority functions
> **S**eek the source of all wisdom
> **S**ensitive to others

These two anonymous sayings are my favorites:

May misfortune follow you all the days of your life . . . and never overtake you.

Labor at prayer and then watch God work.

Prayer: Remind me to prioritize and live my life according to Your direction.

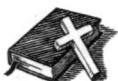

July 23

Are You Dry?

In the last day, that great day of the feast, Jesus stood and cried saying. 'If any man thirst, let him come unto me and drink.
He that believeth on me, as the scripture hath said, out of his belly shall flow rivers of living water. John 2:37,38

One morning I sat on my back patio for time with God away from the distractions of life. There in Texas, we were going through the worst heat wave and drought on the record books. Our summer vacation lasted twelve days. When we returned, our beautiful Saint Augustine grass, my husband's pride and the source of many compliments, was brown and brittle.

Sometimes, that's the way we feel. I've had days when trying to pray took too much energy. My mind flitted to more exciting things. I felt that God was a million miles away. My spirit was parched and unproductive.

My husband watered the grass the night we returned. He continued watering every morning and every evening. The first couple of weeks, we saw no improvement. Then, small green sprouts poked their heads above ground. We fertilized and watered more. Four and a half weeks later, I looked across our back yard and noticed the green overtaking the brown. The lush Saint Augustine reached again toward the hot sun, reviving water and food in its roots.

The same can be true of our spiritual life. Jesus tells us he's the living water. If we become dry, we must go back to adding Jesus to our lives despite our feelings. We must feed our souls with His word and apply water every day or twice a day. With time, we'll stand tall against the heat of trials and temptations because Jesus nourishes our inner selves.

Prayer: I need Your water and food every day else I grow dry and die.

July 24

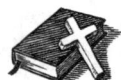

Pride Comes in Many Forms

He hath put down the mighty from their seats, and exalted them of low degree. Luke 1:52

God hates pride—not good self-esteem—but arrogance, egotism, conceit, narcissism. A braggart is one who worships himself instead of his creator.

The Bible tells stories of people who thought more highly of themselves than they should, and God brought them down.

- Pharaoh thought he could outwit God and keep the Israelites working in Egypt, but God sent ten plagues and destroyed his army in the Red Sea.
- Nebuchadnezzar required all the people to bow down to him. He thought he was invincible, but God took his mind and sent him out with the animals.
- Haman built a gallows for God's man but ended up hanging on it himself.

We recognize pride in people who brag and constantly talk about how great they are, but do we see it in the "martyr complex" prevalent in many compulsive overeaters? At my worst, I controlled my whole family by my "woe is me" attitude. I'd burst into tears. My husband could not placate me. My daughters couldn't console. When I didn't get my way, I stormed the house. A cloud fell on everyone's activities. It was all about me and what I wanted.

That's pride, my friend.

Did I say that God hates pride? Pride worsens a compulsive personality. We injure the ones we love the most. We destroy God's work in our lives. The more I refused to surrender my bad attitude, the more I ate compulsively. The cycle never ended until I submitted my pride to Christ.

Prayer: When things don't go my way, may I seek Your way.

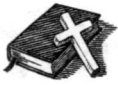

July 25

Criticism Is Gold

Don't refuse to accept criticism, get all the help you can.
Proverbs 23:7 Life Recovery Bible

I guess no one likes criticism but sometimes we need it, and sometimes we need to give it.

Three steps to take before *accepting* criticism:

1. Is the person offering corrective advice a true friend? Do they want what's best for you?
2. Have you prayed about what they told you?
3. Can you incorporate the advice or criticism into your life?

Three steps to take before *giving* criticism:

1. Have you prayed about the criticism you plan to give?
2. Think about your motivation for your comments. Is it pure and unselfish?
3. Are you willing to help the person follow your advice?

No man is an island. Most of us aren't even peninsulas. We need a team of support surrounding us, especially when we set out to change the direction for our lives. Twelve-step meetings, church classes, and other support groups fill this need.

During the last weight class I taught at church, I received advice from two sources. One of them encouraged me, but one made me mad. I took the advice above and prayed about them. I considered the sources and determined how it applied to my life. I needed both things. As the verse says, we need all the help we can get.

Prayer: May I never turn aside criticism that You send and I need.

July 26

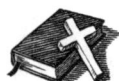

A False God

No man can serve two masters, for either he will hate the one and love the other; or else he will hold to the one, and despise the other. Ye cannot serve God and mammon. Matthew 6:24

The heart of man cries out for God. To satisfy that hunger, many of us turn to false gods. At age seven, I gave my heart to Jesus. Though I backslid from Him in my first year of college, I returned and rededicated my life. While struggling with low self-esteem and depression, instead of allowing God to heal me, I turned to food. Though I didn't realize it for years, I sought help in a false god.

Food hindered a good relationship with my husband and children and kept me from following Christ as He planned. Despite my longing to be what I knew I should be, I failed. My false god led me into deeper and harder battles and almost won the war when I contemplated suicide.

Jesus tried to tell us we can't serve two gods. If food masters our thoughts and actions, then God takes a back seat as the verse explains. It's impossible to be an overeater given to obsessive, compulsive binges and serve God with all your heart.

"Please be aware that Satan will fill your mind (if he is allowed to) with all types of negative thinking about yourself and will build strongholds in your mind." *Battlefield of the Mind* by Joyce Meyer.

Prayer: Fill my mind and help me love the real God with all my heart.

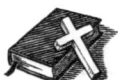

July 27

Something New

A new commandment I give unto you, that ye love one another; as I have loved you, that ye also love one another. John 13:34

Even Jesus tried something new. This wasn't a change in beliefs, but a new method, a new way to look at an old commandment.

God's Ten Commandments given to Moses started with loving and honoring God. He then moved to a) not killing, b) not stealing, c) not lying, and other rules revolving around loving others.

Still upholding the original commandments, Jesus gave a new one—not only should we treat others right, but we should love them.

Giving a problem like compulsive overeating to Jesus isn't a new concept for most of us, but Jesus wants to "give us a new commandment." In other words, He wants you to try something different.

I tried every method known to man to lose weight, but success came when I gave up and quit trying because man's ways didn't work. Try something new:

- If you've been seeking God and then working to make it work, try not working anymore. Try leaving it up to God.
- If you've thought of God as your co-pilot, think of him as the one who's flying the plane with you in the back.
- If you've tried following a rigid diet plan, try not planning your food, but asking Him to choose it daily.
- If you continue to fail at something, do it totally different.
- If you've never read an inspirational book or got devotions every day by e-mail, start now.

Jesus wants to give you a new commandment, a new method, a new outlook.

Prayer: Change my viewpoint today.

July 28

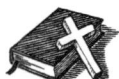

List of Do's and Don'ts

For by grace are ye saved through faith, and that not of yourselves: It is the gift of God. Not of works, lest any man should boast. Ephesians 2:8,9

The Old Testament covenant gave the Israelites ten commandments plus many other rules. The people failed. Following the list required God's power within them. The commands showed them where they erred. God sent leaders, prophets and miracles to demonstrate his love and power. All His people had to do was lean on Him.

We run down the Israelites because of their rebellion and relapse again and again after God worked wonderful works for them. But are we Christians not the same? Even when we've witnessed God's power and experienced His strength, we stumble and falter because we again turn to our own inept abilities.

Diets give us a strict list of dos and don'ts. Eat lettuce and broccoli. Don't eat cake or pizza. Rules and regulations never work for humans, especially those of us with compulsive disorders. When we're told no, we rebel. To know we must avoid candy, we desire it more. When we're told we must exercise thirty minutes a day, our minds resist, our muscles refuse.

We must have absolute faith in God if we are to be absolutely obedient. Henrietta C. Mears

Prayer: I always fail, so help me lean on Your strength.

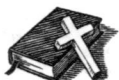

July 29

Pass It on

Don't forget to do good and to share what you have with those in need, for such sacrifices are pleasing to him.
Hebrews 13:16 Life Recovery Bible

In a twelve-step program such as Overeater's Anonymous, the final or twelfth step is to "take the message to others who are suffering."

Paul tells us that same thing in Hebrews. My dad used to always say, "you have to pay your dues." Another familiar saying is "practice what you preach." The first step in following Christ is to entrust your heart to Him and begin walking with Him. So, too, the first step of compulsive overeating health is to entrust the journey to Him and take the first step.

What is your first step?

- Buy healthy foods?
- Join a gym?
- Study inspirational books?

Before you do any of that, before you start the day, PRAY.

After you follow Christ and "keep doing good" as the verse says, then pass it on to others. Encourage another overeater whenever you can. Teach a class. Speak up about what's helped you. Much of our healing is based on us "passing it on." God loves when we witness.

Could it be that, like members of Overeater's Anonymous, our recovery depends on trying to help others?

Prayer: Lead me to someone who needs my encouragement today.

July 30

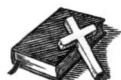

What's Your Up and Down Ratio?

Thou shalt have no other gods before me. Exodus 20:3

God's Word tells us that He's jealous of our love. Jesus says the first and greatest commandment is to love God with everything in us; our strength, our mind, our heart.

In my life, I've noticed this equation in both directions:

- My love of food goes down.
- My love of God goes up.
- I start thinking about food more.
- I start having less thought of Jesus.

God wishes us to put Him first, so food shouldn't even be in our top five list. No, that's not an easy task. At first, we may have to give conscious effort to turn our thoughts aside when food temptations draw us. But the more we obey God in our eating the less food compels. Certain foods serve as magnets. Try reading His word or praying when food seduces. God can and will help.

What is your up and down ratio today? What attracted your mind when you woke? Try waking up to a thanks-to-God prayer. Food then loses its luster.

Prayer: Today I will focus on You more.

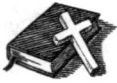

July 31

Persistence Counts

But ye, brethren, be not weary in well doing. 2 Thessalonians 3:13

I will never reach my destination if all I do is start the trip. If I decide to go to Aurora, Colo. to visit my daughter, but I stop in Colorado Springs, I do not reach my goal. Getting closer is admirable, but I do not see my daughter. I don't accomplish what I wanted.

Think back over the reason you started the weight loss journey. Why did you begin reading these daily devotions? Why did you relinquish your will and your food to Christ? In doing this, it's not enough to do it for three months or three years. This is a lifetime battle, a never-ending trip.

Just like our walk in salvation, Jesus encourages us to not grow tired in doing what we know we should do. Practice persistence.

In *Super Thesaurus* by Marc McCutcheon, to *persist* lists synonyms as: persevere, continue, carry on, endure, "stick to it, keep up, be steadfast, hang in there, survive."

I especially like that last one—survive. That's what it takes. Until our dying breath, we travel the road to salvation and submission. We survive.

In our local Weight Watcher pamphlet last week, this quote came out and I put it on my refrigerator:

The people that reach their goal weight aren't perfect, they're persistent.

Prayer: Help me make it one more day.

August 1

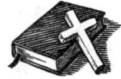

What Is Coming Out of Your Mouth?

Not that which goeth into the mouth defileth a man; but that which cometh out of the mouth, this defileth a man.
Matthew 15:11.

Yes, eating candy, donuts and Big Macs will make you obese, but what you put into your mouth is not the root or cause of your trouble. Jesus tells us that out of our hearts comes bad things which include greed, quarrels, adultery and gluttony.

I know you're thinking that gluttony comes from putting extra food in your mouth. But overeating is a sign that something is wrong inside your heart.

A saying enclosed in my order of Guidepost greeting cards says, "Holding onto anger is like grasping a hot coal with the intent of throwing it at someone else. You are the one who gets burned."

Let's put this into perspective with other problems besides anger:

- If we're the ones who hold onto resentment, we're the ones who succumb to bitterness and become hateful personalities, the ones nobody likes.
- If we associate with evil men because of greed, we reap the consequences when they come for our lives.
- If we obstinately refuse to give up a certain food, we're the ones who get fat and encounter prejudice.

Don't worry so much about what diet you follow (what you put into your mouth), worry about your relationship with the Lord (what comes out of your mouth).

Prayer: I love You, Lord, with all my heart.

213

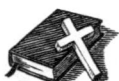

August 2

What's Ahead?

For to be carnally minded is death; but to be spiritually minded is life and peace. Romans 8:6

God is prepared for anything that might happen to us.

Peace eludes us when we worry. I used to start bingeing on food at the first thought that something bad might happen. By the time the worst struck, I was drowning in compulsive over-eating and no longer in control of my emotions. In a short time, I spiraled into depression. Too much food tranquilized my thought processes so that I couldn't cope with the smallest dilemma.

What worries you masters you. Haddon W. Robinson

If we begin today to focus on Christ, our problems ease, our minds relax, and our coping-mechanisms engage.

If we concentrate on what we might eat, our problems increase, our minds becomes depressed, and our coping-powers are non-existent.

Jesus provides peace and hope and joy to those who seek it in Him. To what are you looking to alleviate your worries?

Prayer: May my faith destroy my worry.

August 3

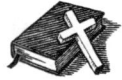

Clear Skies

With long life will I satisfy him; and shew him my salvation.
Psalms 91:16

This morning I sat on my back patio and viewed the clearness of the sky. With the extreme drought and hot temperatures this summer, fires threaten on every side of our city. Last night, ashes floated through the air and dusted our hair and clothing. Winds calmed through the night and this morning, our sky is a crystal expanse of sapphire.

God showed me how that was also true of my view of life. When we were younger and raising our daughters, disorder drove my deductive reasoning. I loved Jesus, but focusing on myself distorted my view of His direction for my life.

We sing a song at church titled "It's All About Him." As a young adult, life was all about me. I was mistreated. I couldn't stop craving sweets, but they made me fat. It wasn't fair. My husband traveled and left me to handle everything. I tired of arguing with my girls, so I had to eat. I did more at church than Sister So-and-so, but she got the praise.

Sound familiar?

Every age offers good and bad. Now, I lament being so old and having a shorter time to accomplish all I want to do. But, now that God controls all of me, I liken the older ages to my clear sky this morning. I see Your hand in everything. As the psalmist said, He shows us His salvation. He never leaves us. But, sometimes our view is covered with ashes.

Prayer: Remove the ash and help me see clearly.

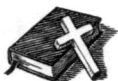

August 4

Failure

Be of good courage, and he shall strengthen your heart, all ye that hope in the Lord. Psalms 31:24

I prepare the feast
With heavy heart.
Faults bog me down
Fear sets me apart.

I stir the foods, but
Something's not right.
My hands shake
As I take a bite.

I taste bitterness for sure.
What's that ingredient?
Submission to God makes
Giving in expedient.

I bow before the heavenly throne
Knowing I'm unworthy.
On my own, I fall short
Cling to food that's earthly.

I've worked for You,
I plead with God.
Did I misread Your command?
I want You to applaud.

(Poem continued tomorrow)

Prayer: When I am weak and fail, remind me, You're at Your strongest.

August 5

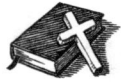

Success

For whatsoever is born of God overcometh the world; and this is the victory that overcometh the world, even our faith. 1 John 5:4

(Poem continued from yesterday)

No, my child He explains.
You don't know my thoughts
They're higher than yours
So don't be distraught.

Dessert will come later.
I view the whole meal.
Stay in the kitchen
Pray for the yield.

How say you, you've failed
When the dinner's not ready.
The yeast is still rising
Now hold fast and steady.

At banquet time
I'll sound the alert.
We'll gather round the table
In me, you'll have worth.

By Janet K. Brown

Prayer: In Jesus, I have great worth regardless of my size.

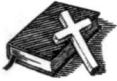

August 6

Sacrifice Your Will

And so, dear brothers, I plead with you to give your bodies to God,
Let them be a living sacrifice, holy—the kind he can accept.
When you think of what he has done for you, is this too much to
ask? Romans 12:1 Life Recovery Bible

The clash of wills goes on endlessly. In Scripture, even Paul
tells us he does what he doesn't want to do and doesn't do what
he wants to. God calls on us to be holy and acceptable to Him.
As sinners, He loves us. As failures, He picks us up from the
ditch.

Yet, the call remains: "Give your bodies as living sacrifices."
God expects imperfection. He accepts us as we are. He offers
His shoulder to lean on, His footsteps to guide and His strength
when ours gives way to weakness.

If we don't give up our wills, we fall into blaming other
people or situations. When we play the blame games, we open
our minds to Satan's lies. Then, we build resentment and try to
eliminate hurt feelings with food.

Jesus expects us to daily sacrifice our will. We place our will
in subjection to His when we pray, "Let my will, my choices, my
life be Yours." We mustn't ask Him to always sacrifice His will
because He loves us. Think what He's already done. He took
man's place on the cross. Is it too much to daily die to what
foods we desire to keep a closer relationship with Him?

Today, let's think of Jesus' sacrifice and then measure our
own. Do they balance?

Prayer: Lord, kill my will today.

August 7

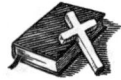

Potential

Don't copy the behavior and customs of this world, but be a new and different person with a fresh newness in all you do and think. Then, you will learn from your own experience how his ways will really satisfy you. Romans 12:2 Life Recovery Bible

We hold great potential for excellence.

After the reference yesterday, we continue to read the next verse in Romans today. Let us dwell on our potential for change. With God's help, it's enormous.

As children, my three daughters sang a song that goes, "I am a promise, I am a possibility." I always loved that thought. However, at two hundred and fifty pounds with low self-esteem, I failed to see any potential worth in myself.

The above verse gives hope to those without any resources left. How many times I had wished for a new body, a new beginning, a new plan, but try as I might, every beginning ended the same way—back in the same hole with more weight than I'd had before. Time to try something different, like giving up.

If we never thought about food today, what could we accomplish?

- Teach a class
- Write a book
- Visit shut-ins

Create your own list. Our potentials in Christ are limitless.

Prayer: Mold me into the vision You have for my life today.

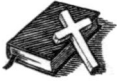

August 8

Praise the Lord and pass His food.

Which executeth judgment for the oppressed; which giveth food to the hungry, The Lord looseth the prisoners. The Lord openeth the eyes of the blind; the Lord raiseth them that are bowed down; the Lord loveth the righteous Psalms 146:7, 8

Our relationship with the Lord is a private meal; it's never a feast with friends.

Study the above verse with care. What does it promise?

1. God judges our enemies.
2. God provides spiritual and physical nourishment.
3. God sets captives free.
4. God helps us see truth.
5. God encourages those of us depressed.
6. God loves us.

Now, that's quite a banquet table for one.

In an old book of my mother's entitled "KIXL's Think-it-Overs," I like this quote. "Faith must be always the big brother of hope . . . guarding that rather delicate youngster from the attacks of the bullies of the mind . . . the fears and threats and doubts which are ambushed in life."

As the title of the book suggests, "think it over."

God provides everything we need, but we need faith to access hope, and faith comes from God, too.

Prayer: Your table provides everything I require to succeed.

August 9

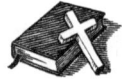

I Already Pray. Why Meditate?

Meditate upon these things; give thyself wholly to them; that thy profiting may appear to all. 1 Timothy 4:15

In a twelve-step program, step eleven urges participants to pray and meditate. Several scriptures, such as the one above, insist we meditate.

What's the difference?

Definitions from Webster's New World Dictionary are:

Pray—to implore, petition, or ask

Meditate—to think deeply, to ponder

So, prayer means we ask God for something, and meditate means we give Him time to talk to us.

As a child, the Biblical Samuel lived and worked with Eli, the priest. One night, Samuel answered the call of the Holy Spirit by saying "Speak, Lord for thy servant heareth;" (1 Samuel 3:9)

Today, much interferes with our hearing. How many times have we knelt to pray and battled other thoughts? The Word specifies prayer and meditation—not either/or—because we need both.

In one class I learned to first praise God before asking for anything. The reason for this is we focus our attention on Him and how wonderful He is.

I focus on God. I think on Him. I listen to Him. How else can He direct my food choices in the proper way? And that's His part.

God does His part well, but "letting go" is a choice we make daily.

Prayer: May I make time for prayer and meditation today.

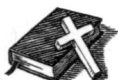

August 10

Be Alert and Vigilant

Fight the good fight of faith, lay hold on eternal life; whereunto thou are also called and have professed a good profession before many witnesses. 1 Timothy 6:12

With a line of other children, I marched into church for the convening of Vacation Bible School feeling as if I'd enlisted in God's army. We studied Bible warriors Joshua and David. We learned the strong stands of Daniel and Ezekiel. Teachers armed us with the necessary weaponry. Each child, including me, yearned to fight for Christ.

Song leaders in our church peppered our Sunday music with militant Christian melodies. The titles of our hymns included 'A Mighty Fortress is our God," "Onward Christian Soldiers" and "Stand Up for Jesus, Ye Soldiers of the Cross." Who could forget the Christian song that became a theme of the civil war, "The Battle Hymn of the Republic"?

The spirit of reformation framed previous congregations as a mighty fighting force. I think in America, where life is too easy for some, we've lost some of that vigilance. As a recovering compulsive overeater, I must remain alert and prepared for battle. Just because I've succeeded for years doesn't mean the devil will leave me alone. Like an Army general does, Satan plans a new strategy or a new direction for attack.

To follow Christ, I must keep the spirit of the militant, triumphant church of old and march into battle daily.

Prayer: Today, help me "fight the good fight."

August 11

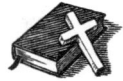

Use It or Lose It

And thine ears shall hear a word behind thee saying: This is the way; walk ye in it, when ye turn to the right hand, and when ye turn to the left. Isaiah 30:21

We took each step toward healing.

1. We admitted we were powerless over food.
2. We gave up and asked God to take our will, our choices, our lives.
3. We prayed and asked God to show us problem areas.
4. We meditate on God.

What now? How do we know what to do on a daily basis? Do those things above every day.
I like this quote from *Thoughts for All Seasons*.

There is a law that seems to work. Use it or lose it. You must use your muscles or lose your power. You must walk or you will lose the ability to walk. You must use your voice or lose it. Some of you can throw a ball straight and true now, but ten years from now, you will not be able to unless you keep on using your throwing arm.

We must walk the path with God and use our faith muscle, or we won't be able to refrain from compulsiveness again. Use the power, or no longer be able to access it.

Prayer: For this new day, help me hear You speak. Infuse me with faith.

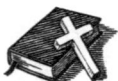

August 12

Out of Ashes

Wherefore I abhor myself and repent in dust and ashes. So, the Lord blessed the latter end of Job more than his beginning.
Job 42:6, 12a

A few years ago, my husband and I went through a difficult time in our church. Though we had prayed much over the choice of a new pastor and voted to call a certain man, we were disappointed. He immediately ran many of us off with personal attacks interwoven with misinterpreted theology. We and many other families dispersed across the city into other churches. Two former members called us to talk about a meeting to discuss the problem.

The afternoon meeting found three hundred people hungry for the Word of God and a place to worship. We were blown away by the movement of God in our midst. A new church was born that day. Now, after ten years, God blesses both the new and the old church.

During this time, my husband and I spotted a work of art by Jesse Barnes, an artist who uses light in special ways. We purchased a picture entitled "Out of Ashes." It frames a new world coming to life in the light of a bright flame of fire. That picture hangs over our mantel and often speaks to me.

Today, when I falter, when I am fatigued, frustrated, and fraught with anxiety, God directs my eyes to that painting. Eighteen years ago, my life was a heap of ashes. I felt empty and void of peace. God raised up beauty from that and is blessing me more than He did in the beginning.

Remember, always, where you came from then God will lead you to the future He has planned.

Prayer: Thank You for lifting me out of ashes and helping me daily.

August 13

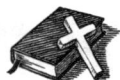

In the Day

In the day when I cried thou answeredst me, and strengthenedst me with strength in my soul. Psalms 138:3

What's your day like today? Do you feel strong or weak? Are you running errands, working or housecleaning? Are you in town or out of town?

Are you eating healthy or eating everything in sight?

From the book *Celebration of Discipline* by Richard J. Foster, I read this: "We do not want to be beginners. But let us be convinced of the fact that we will never be anything else but beginners all our life." He's referring to focusing on God through certain disciplines and letting God take over our besetting sins.

Though I've walked this journey for eighteen years, I find this is true. Today, I started out ready to give up and binge on favorite foods. I began weak and ended strong. Why? Because in my weakness, I cried out to God.

The lyrics of a song by Don Moen called "Give Thanks" advise: "Let the weak say I am strong, let the poor say I am rich." I love that song. I "give thanks" today for the truth of those words.

Prayer: Thank You, Lord, that this beginner still gains strength from You regardless of what this day offers.

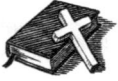

August 14

Thank You

Give thanks to the Lord, call on his name; make known among the nations what he has done. 1 Chronicles 16:8 NIV

During my quiet time today, my heart filled with praise. I couldn't petition the Lord for anything new. All I could do was say "thank You." From that spring of gratitude, I wrote this little verse.

I stand in awe of Your majesty.
I'm overwhelmed by Your power.
Help me be all that I can be
Since You pulled me out of the mire.

Blessed be Thy name, Dear Lord.
My hands rise up in praise.
Let me not fail to hear Your Word
And honor You all my days.

Have you ever felt like writing a poem to God or singing a song? Wouldn't that be a good thing to do today?

Prayer: You've done so much for me. Sometimes, all I can do is say "thank You."

August 15

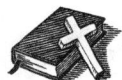

Growing or Swelling

Better it is to be of an humble spirit with the lowly than to divide the spoil with the proud. Proverbs 16:19

It should never be all about me.

My lifetime of martyr complexes was pride.

Deliver me from pride, and give me a humble spirit.

Years ago, after my oldest daughter's wedding, anger drove me to days of wallowing in self-pity. Pride and humiliation ruined a special day for me.

Old friends didn't come to the wedding. I carried resentment toward them for years. With God's emotional healing, I let go that resentment and learned to love them again.

When I get hot and anxious, my cheeks flare with heat, turning them scarlet. At the wedding, friends asked about my red face, if I had blood pressure problems. I didn't at that time, but I resented the suggestion. I saw those comments the same as asking if my being fat gave me health troubles. I seethed in silence and remained in bed for four days after my daughter and new son-in-law left on their honeymoon. God's healing focused my attention on Him and gave me a proper perspective toward my friends.

Since God healed me and set me on a path to weight loss and intimacy with Christ, I remember those days and realize my anger stemmed from pride. Life was all about me. Now I concentrate on God and pride dissipates.

"Some people grow under responsibility; others swell." From *Thought for All Seasons* by Henrietta C. Mears

Prayer: May I allow God to help me grow and live with a lowly, humble spirit.

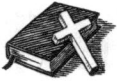

August 16

Give Me a Token

Bind them continually upon thine heart and tie them about thy neck. Proverbs 6:21

God knew the importance of remembering. Throughout Scripture, symbols are given to help believers remember. In the Old Testament, blood on the doorpost and eating Passover meals reminded the Israelites of God's deliverance from the Egyptians. In the New Testament, Jesus instituted the taking of the bread and wine in remembrance of His sacrifice.

In all areas of life, tokens or mementos remind us of something important that we wish to not forget. At a Weight Watcher meeting years ago, the teacher advised us to use a token or some sort of memory so we don't forget where we started. At that time, I had lost much of my weight and wore a pair of red shorts I liked after years of them setting in my closet. They fit like second skin, but I could get them on. As I lost more and more, I felt the waistband loosen until I could pull it way out from my waist. That evolved into a token for me. Even today, I pull out the waist of those red shorts, and I envision when I cried over the rolls of fat that kept them from getting over my torso. I thank God for the miracle He gave me.

After attending Overeaters Anonymous, I purchased a coin with the OA insignia and the motto "One day at a time" engraved on it. I carried it for years as a token of my success. When I look at it, I relive that slogan.

Today, choose for yourself a verse of Scripture or a token of some sort to remind you of where you were and where you're going.

Prayer: I will hide Your Word in my heart today as a token of Your faithfulness.

August 17

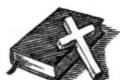

Deceit is Sneaky

But have renounced the hidden things of dishonesty, not walking in craftiness, nor handling the word of God deceitfully but by manifestation of the truth, commending ourselves to every man's conscience in the sight of God. 2 Corinthians 4:2

You can't obtain true intimacy without complete truth, and God can't heal you if deceit remains. God requires no less than your full heart, no more than complete honesty.

If we dissect the above verse, notice the things to get rid of: Hidden things — Craftiness — Dishonesty — Deceit

The hardest thing for me to do is buy a favorite food and eat it while someone comments: "You're going to eat that whole bag?" But, God requires that of me. If I eat it, I can't hide it.

I was always a closet eater. As soon as everyone left, I took my candy from the back of the pantry or the bottom of my drawer (hidden things) and ate it all before they returned. I ate normal-sized meals with my family, saying I wasn't hungry, (deceit) when actually, my stomach felt sick from overeating. My husband would ask if I still had that ten dollar bill he gave me just in case, and I would say, "No, I had to buy a card for Mom." I spent $1.50 on Mom and $8 for candy and donuts (dishonesty). I hid the candy in the glove compartment until my husband went into the back yard and then I snuck it into my sock drawer .(craftiness)

Those of us plagued with compulsive personalities obsess over having both worlds. We want Christ to help us eat better. But we play games. Surely we can binge-eat occasionally?

Is that not "handling the word of God" deceitfully? I must be open and above board about anything I eat. God will heal what we give to Him, open and with no sneaky business.

Prayer: Let my life be open to Your healing touch.

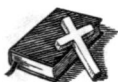

August 18

I've Failed Too Many Times

This I recall to my mind; therefore I hope. It is of the Lord's mercies that we are not consumed, because his compassions fail not. They are new every morning; great is thy faithfulness.
Lamentations 3:21-23

When I read this verse, all I can say is "Hallelujah. Praise the Lord."

In the beginning, my mind tormented me with my failure. I remembered the times I shouted at my kids because they interrupted me with a bag of Reese's. My bad mood came from embarrassment that I'd been caught. I remembered the times I hastened my husband out the door because the snack in the pantry called my name. I recalled times of new beginnings to be followed by greater defeats. I agree with Jeremiah that it was a wonder I wasn't consumed for my faithlessness.

When I started this last journey to healing, God showed me this verse to remember. For every one of my failures, God's mercies extended farther. Every time I fell on my face, God's compassion lifted me in love.

I've failed so many times it is no longer an excuse. How can I ever fail more than God can heal with grace, mercy and love?

Here is a brief sketch of Abraham Lincoln's life:

1831 – Failed in business
1832 – Defeated for Legislature
1833 – Defeated for Elector
1843 – Defeated for Congress
1848 – Defeated for Senate
1855 – Defeated for Vice President
1860 – Elected President of the United States!

KIXL's "Think-It-Overs"

Prayer: Praise God for mercies that supersede defeat.

230

August 19

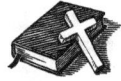

I'm Only a Bridge

Let not your heart be troubled; ye believe in God, believe also in me. John 14:1

Too many times, we face the future with trepidation. The flood of work we have to do or the problems soon to be faced overwhelms us. If we leaned on our own power, we would be right to despair. We can't handle it. We grow in desire to hide or run to a deserted island where trouble can't find us. Our emotions run aground.

The phrase "one day at a time" is a good slogan to remember. As the old Chinese proverb states, "A trip of a thousand miles begins with the first step." Memorize the Scripture above and quote it when you see an avalanche headed your way.

Another good quote is:

"Man, like the bridge, was designed to carry the load of the moment, not the combined weight of a year at once." William A. Ward.

Focus on one moment at a time.

Memorize the above verse.

Take one baby step at a time.

Look up to heaven.

Prayer: Lord, remind me today that You created me like a bridge.

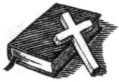

August 20

Make a Decision

For I the Lord thy God will hold thy right hand, saying unto thee. Fear not, I will help thee. Isaiah 41:13

Many things in life require a choice. Somewhere along the way, you chose a college, a spouse, or a job. Think about the process of making a decision important to your life. What does it involve? For a Christian, prayer may come first. Then, what?

The verse above brought about an important decision for me six years ago. For two years, my husband and I had gone back and forth on the idea of me retiring from my demanding job as a bookkeeper and insurance coder for a doctor's office. I would be ready to quit, but my husband would pose reasons for delaying. Then, we flip-flopped. He'd want me to quit, but I thought it not wise. During this time, many prayers went up for guidance. Three times, we made a list of pros and cons then decided the cons overruled the pros, so I kept working.

One night, my troubled mind kept me awake. We wanted to take two of our grandchildren to San Antonio for spring break, but being in different schools, they were out on different weeks. I couldn't take off for vacation both weeks without giving up our summer plans. You can believe I prayed a lot while I lay awake. My granddaughter was thirteen. If I waited until I planned on retirement three years later, she might not want to go with me. The next morning, I awoke with a surety that retirement at that moment was right. I opened my Bible starting with David Wilkerson's verse for the day. I read Isaiah 41:13, and I knew. We never regretted that decision.

Committing your eating to God is a decision:

Pray—List pros and cons—Step out in faith.

Prayer: Thank You for helping me with the decision to give in to Your will today.

August 21

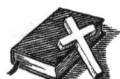

Pick Up Your Prize

Know ye not that they which run in a race run all, but one receiveth the prize? So run, that ye may obtain.
1 Corinthians 9:14

When I enter a contest or run a race, I want to win. Don't you? But every day, misguided people waste money on lottery tickets, hoping to win. As Paul reminds us, only one can win a race. But, look at his inspired advice: "Run, that ye may obtain." Put your best into everything you do—work, play, worship, eating. Everything.

Still, a few prizes or gifts along the way help encourage us to stretch for a goal. I've been told that it takes twenty-one days to make a new habit. Should we not receive a reward for committing a difficult problem, like compulsive overeating, over to God for twenty-one days?

I remember several landmark awards along my path:

- The first time I entered a regular-sized department of women's clothes and bought a dress for church.
- The first time I slipped into a skinny booth at a restaurant and ordered a dessert without guilt.
- The day I ordered a token saying "one day at a time" and knew it was a life-long motto for me.

Surprise yourself with a prize along the way. Don't wait until you reach any magic number on the scale. Do it because you've reached your goal of surrendering your compulsion to Christ. Maybe today is a day for a reward.

Prayer: An intimate chat with Jesus is today's reward. I thank You.

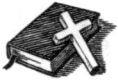

August 22

I Need More Love

One morning, in a Beth Moore Bible study, I prayed for more love for God. His love is overpowering to us, but what about our love of Him. He answered me. Today, all I can do is focus on Jesus.

The Lord is my shepherd; I shall not want.
He maketh me to lie down in green pastures; he leadeth me beside the still waters.
He restoreth my soul; he leadeth me in the paths of righteousness for his name's sake
Yea, though I walk through the valley of the shadow of death, I will fear no evil; for thou art with me, thy road and thy staff they comfort me.
Thou preparest a table before me in the presence of mine enemies; thou anointest my head with oil; my cup runneth over.
Surely goodness and mercy shall follow me all the days of my life; and I will dwell in the house of the Lord for ever.
Psalms 23: 1-6

If you don't already know those verses, memorize them. Say them every night and every morning. How great is God. How worthy of our love. Seek Him first and the love of food dissipates.

Prayer: Thank You, Lord. I love You.

August 23

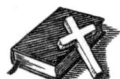

Relax and Be happy

A relaxed attitude lengthens a man's life; jealousy rots it away.
Proverbs 14:20 Life Recovery Bible

Some years ago, a song became popular with the theme "Relax. Be happy." This song meant eating, drinking, partying. Christians have a better right to relax and be happy than anyone. The partying crowd worries about a hangover the morning after or weight gain from uninhibited gluttony. When we walk with Christ, worries roll onto His shoulders. We no longer have to lug them on our backs.

Now focus on the second part of that proverb about jealousy. Years of jealousy, resentment and anger drove me to worship at the idol of eating. I desired sweeter snacks and more indulgence to cover the mental instabilities. The wisdom of the Proverbs describes this as "rotting me away," and so it did.

Could it be that a relaxed attitude lengthening our lives is merely another way God reminds us of the ravages of sin? While I ate more and more, Satan ate away at my faith.

Prayer: Today, I desire to relax and be happy in God.

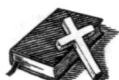

August 24

No Put-Downs

He that believeth on him is not condemned; but he that believeth not is condemned already, because he hath not believed in the name of the only begotten Son of God. John 3:18

God doesn't put us down. When we believe on Jesus, He brings no condemnation, no guilt. He deals with us as wayward, but loved, children.

Who is it that condemns you?

- Friends?
- Spouse?
- Prospective bosses?

Many of these ridicule or show prejudice to overweight people. Yet the worst culprit for condemnation comes from ourselves. Satan uses this against us. He whispers in our ears that we might as well give up. We're hopeless. We've turned our backs on God, so He will turn His on us.

Lies

Lies

Lies

He that believeth on Christ is not condemned. The Holy Spirit points out areas we need to improve, but He never loads guilt. His dealing is gentle as a baby's breath, as soft as the touch of a slight breeze.

No more put-downs from you.

Never any put-downs from God.

Overcome the world as He overcame it.

Prayer: I shed all guilt because it doesn't come from You.

August 25

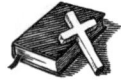

In the Battle

His work will be shown for what it is, because the day will bring it to light. It will be revealed with fire, and the fire will test the quality of each man's work. If what he has built survives, he will receive his reward; if it is burned up, he will suffer loss . . .
1 Corinthians 3:13,14 NIV

Examples abound to show us how God uses struggle to refine and improve. The battle makes us strong. Today, see how many examples you can think of where struggles improved the situation.

Look at a baby who learns to walk. With great effort, he pulls himself up to a table. Then, he gets the nerve to let go his security. After one or two steps, he falls. He sits and cries. However, in no time, he tries again, and again, and again. The process strengthens the baby's legs and finally he walks across the room. Struggles propel the child forward.

Look at the pearl. The oyster has two separate shells. When a foreign body gets in the middle, a substance is secreted to cover it. So, a pearl forms from a foreign substance covered up, but continually irritated. The irritation makes a beautiful gem.

Look at the metamorphosis of the caterpillar. The insect crawls onto a leaf and pulls a covering over himself for protection. Inside, changes occur until the new body grows stronger. When mighty enough, he breaks through the chrysalis (or covering) with wet wings that don't fly, but the built-up strength causes him to take flight an hour later.

When you think it's too hard to conquer your compulsion, remember the struggle makes you stronger. You're in the war to win. Keep up the fight. The reward belongs to those who complete the race. Look up. Your deliverance has come.

Prayer: I'll fight one more day with Your help.

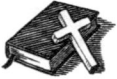

August 26

Get in Your Conflict

Be sober, be vigilant; because your adversary the devil, as a roaring lion, walketh about seeking whom he may devour.
1 Peter 5:8

I know all about conflict in my stories. I mostly write fiction. My main character needs a goal, a motivation and a conflict. Why does a fictional hero need conflict?

In the craft of writing, that's called the character's arc. The character's belief starts as one thing, he goes through certain points (conflicts) in the story, and comes out with a revised outlook. That's growth.

God desires we grow in Him. Conflict becomes the mode of growth. When given one conflict, we adjust what we want from life. Another comes along and changes us more. If we avoid conflict at all costs, we impede our growth.

Don't fear the conflict or the battles, welcome them as challenges. Thank God for them. Each setback or failure grants us more insight to better equip us for the next battle.

"If I find myself in a situation of conflict today, I will try working through it rather than attempting to avoid it." *Inner Harvest* by Elizabeth L.

Prayer: Thank You for conflict and stay by my side.

August 27

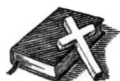

Trumpet Vines and Faithfulness

For the word of the Lord is right and true; he is faithful in all he does. Psalms 33:4 NIV

My husband hates our neighbor's trumpet vines. Three times, Charles tore them off our fence and took them to the dump, but three times, they grew back from the other side. They make him mad because they destroy our wood fence, and he can't dig up the roots to stop the invasion.

This dry summer I studied those vines. The correct name is *campsis radicans*, but most people call them trumpet vines because of the shape of the flowers, like tiny trumpets. Blooms grow up and down each leafy shoot. Ours comes out a vivid orange. Hummingbirds love them. Bees frequent them. Even birds find them enticing. They require minimal soil and love our hot Texas sunshine. When everything, including grass and trees, withered in a hundred days of over a hundred degree temperatures, those trumpet vines still brought color to our backyard.

In considering those vines, I thought of God's faithfulness. Despite good or bad circumstance, God desires to bloom in our lives. He stands ready and able to give us beauty out of ashes, hope out of despair, and growth despite trials. Trumpet vines remind me of God. (Except with no fence destruction).

The next time we face trouble—and we will—think about those beautiful orange blooms that keep giving and giving. That's what God does—he gives eternally.

Prayer: Thank You, Lord, for the reminder today of Your faithfulness.

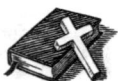

August 28

It's Not Fair

And Joseph said unto them, Fear not, for am I in the place of God?
But as for you, ye thought evil against me, but God meant it unto
good, to bring to pass, as it is this day, to save much people alive.
Genesis 50:19.20

My oldest daughter wisely said that we spend years teaching our children to be fair to others but, by the time they reach the teens, we have to back up and explain that life isn't fair. Perhaps our training as children to be fair is what makes the second lesson far too hard to grasp. If we're fair, why do unfair things happen to us?

God gives marvelous examples in His Word to help us understand this principal. God kicked out the devil from heaven. That cunning ex-angel torments us and foments unrest by sending unjust, unfair happenings on all mankind. For a prescribed time, God allows this to continue even on His children. Yet, when we put these things in God's hands, He brings about good through the bad.

Joseph is a perfect example. He walked with God in uprightness and integrity, but again and again, bad things ensued.

If we allow the bitterness of spirit from it's-not-fair mentality, we don't allow God to illuminate His plans in our lives. The next time I catch myself saying those words, I plan on turning it around. "How exciting to see how God will get me out of this jam once more."

Prayer: Though life's not fair, You're in control and that's all I
need.

August 29

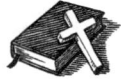

Good News

How beautiful on the mountains are the feet of those who bring good news, who proclaim peace, who bring good tidings, who proclaim salvation, who say to Zion 'Your God reigns!'
Isaiah 52:7

Don't you just want to shout "Hallelujah?"

Yesterday, we returned from a Colorado trip. The beauty and majesty of the mountains remind me of God's might and power. God likened the feet of those bearing the message of hope with the beauty of mountains.

I entitled my online blog "Writing with Hope." My goal is to write stories that give hope in seemingly impossible situations and addictions. Once I faced a load of guilt and a mountain of failures. God sent me the good tidings that He is able and willing to save me from food addiction and all my resentments, envies, and turmoil.

Those glorious mountains bring our problems down to manageable proportions. How small they seem in the light of God's grandeur.

Prayer: Thank You, Lord, for the reminder of Your power in my weakness—good news indeed.

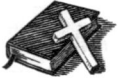

August 30

Difference

Now there are diversities of gifts, but the same Spirit: And there are differences of administrations, but the same Lord. And there are diversities of operations, but it is the same God which worketh all in all. 1 Corinthians 12:4-6

Spending a week with my daughter and son-in-law in Colorado gave me opportunity to study the personalities of their two dogs. Strange, dogs are so different, just like people.

Molly, a standard poodle, is gracious, reserved and easy-going. My daughter tells her something once and Molly obeys. She prefers nibbling her food and spacing it out over hours. She loves to explore the outdoors but rarely barks at other dogs or animals. Left alone, she sleeps and awaits my daughter eagerly with a wave of her tail.

Boo, a Basenji mix, is high-strung, destructive, and gets mad easily. She gulps a bowl of food in seconds and would eat until she was sick if allowed. She loves to play and when she does, she gets very excited and calms slowly. She prefers indoors but when she goes outside, she barks then attacks everything that moves. If you leave her inside alone, she will destroy something.

This story of contrast and the above verse points out our differences. We mustn't allow others to tell us how to walk a spiritual journey to weight loss and maintenance. God's Word will be a light to us. Seek Him. Just as my daughter treats her two dogs in a different manner according to their individual traits, so we need to follow diverse paths to weight loss and emotional healing.

Suggestions from others might be helpful, but get your instruction from God.

Prayer: I'm listening for Your voice, your direction for today.

August 31

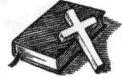

All God's Creatures Need the Light

The Lord is my light and my salvation; whom shall I fear?
The Lord is the strength of my life; of whom shall I be afraid?
Psalms 27:1

As autumn nears, I'm reminded why we have the beautiful changing colors of the season.

Plants use sunlight to turn water and carbon dioxide into oxygen and glucose. This process is called photosynthesis. That means, "putting together with light." Leaves hold a chemical substance named chlorophyll that makes the photosynthesis possible. As summer ends and winter nears, days shorten. As the light lessens, the chlorophyll disappears, leaving leaves without any green. In spring and summer, the green over-whelms the natural color of gold, red or brown. With less light and no green, those colors shine forth until freezing weather causes leaves to drop.

This scientific lesson makes me think of myself. In my own nature, I'm selfish, resentful and generally a mess, but God's sunlight overcomes my shortcomings and puts me together with His light to turn me into something beautiful.

All God's creatures need the Light.

Prayer: Thank You for the light that illuminates my hope.

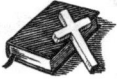

September 1

Drugged

Beloved, I wish above all things that thou mayest prosper and be in health, even as thy soul prospereth. 3 John 2

God desires us to be healthy physically, mentally and spiritually. When we drug ourselves, whether it's with narcotics, alcohol, or food, we cease to be healthy. God can medicate us with peace, love, and hope so that all parts of us prosper.

I desire to be:

> **M**otivated
> **E**ducated
> **D**irected
> **I**nspired
> **C**ommitted
> **A**westruck
> **T**rusting
> **E**ncouraged
> **D**evoted
>
> By God.

Drugged with food? Medicated by God?
Which are you?

Prayer: Physical health as well as spiritual health comes through Jesus.

September 2

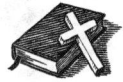

Turning My Turmoil into Hope

Peace, I leave with you, my peace I give unto you; not as the world giveth, give I unto you. Let not your heart be troubled, neither let it be afraid. John 14:27

From my journal:

"I left off my stairs so I could dig into my chocolate covered cherries quicker. I ate a box of twelve, then a package of eight squares of divinity. I finished this before ten and sat my package of miniature Reese's candy in my desk drawer. All day I unwrapped and popped one by one into my mouth . . . . After dinner at home, I crashed. I cared about nothing. I was disgusted with myself."

What a contrast to this excerpt from Isaiah 61:3 NIV:

(The Spirit of the Sovereign Lord is on me) to comfort all who mourn, and provide for those who grieve in Zion—to bestow on them a crown of beauty instead of ashes, the oil of gladness instead of mourning, and a garment of praise instead of a spirit of despair.

My journal continues the next day when I asked for help and leaned on God. Those words sound different:

"I'm one bite away from bondage to food. God must come first. I cannot take it lightly."

Now, I read the words of my journal and think, "Who wrote that?" God has turned my ashes of total despair and desperate food binges into the beauty of praise and hope.

Prayer: I daily open my mind to You to be healed by Your touch.

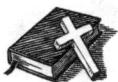

September 3

Love With Action

Dear children, let us not love with words or tongue, but with actions, and in truth. 1 John 3:18 NIV

One of my mother's favorite sayings is: "Actions speak louder than words." How easy to spout that we need to rely on God, but how much harder to turn down a fattening treat when you're all by yourself? Do we think God doesn't see?

> A word with God
> A step of action
> A simple prayer,
> Then, a walk of faith.
> Solitude/ God-brought direction
> Step out then a fraction.
> No way, it's all talk
> Choose the election
> Listen and walk
> Follow, don't balk
> Two components
> For true satisfaction.
>   Janet K. Brown

Pray, but buy healthy foods. Listen, but throw out tempting treats. Study God's word and follow His precepts. Remember, it takes both components for peace, success, and satisfaction.

Prayer: I'll follow where You lead today.

September 4

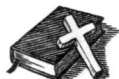

The Eagerness of Heidi

But for you who revere my name, the sun of righteousness will rise with healing in its wings. And you will go out and leap like calves released from the stall. Malachi 4:2 NIV

Our oldest daughter loved horses. When she turned ten, my husband purchased a mare. Julia loved that horse. Heidi was a giant pet. As long as you fed her, she trotted the pastureland with the worrisome load of a ten-year-old trying to be a cowgirl. Our yard wouldn't accommodate this pet, so we stabled her on land a mile or two away from our house. Julia and her father drove every day with a bucket of oats. Before they turned onto the road leading to the pasture, Heidi barreled toward the gate, jumping with excitement.

We see Heidi's action in the above verse. God's healing amazes us. We stand in awe when we remember the past. With God's healing in our wings (heart), we jump with excitement. Food takes its proper place. God is on the throne of our heart. Praise be to Jesus!

Prayer: Thank You, Lord, again and again.

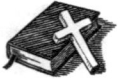

September 5

Even if You're Bad

Don't be frightened, Samuel reassured them. You have certainly done wrong, but make sure now that you worship the Lord with true enthusiasm, and that you don't turn your back on him in any way. Other gods can't help you. The Lord will not abandon his chosen people, for that would dishonor his great name . . .
1 Samuel 12:20-22a, Life Recovery Bible

In the lives of compulsive overeaters, we become emotionally-imbalanced adults. We live selfish lives. We put food and our own petty needs on the throne of our hearts. As we rid our physical bodies of the sugar and fat, our minds clear, and we see ourselves in truth. Guilt overwhelms us. We can't undo the past, but living with the anger, resentment and envy we brought into our families lies like boulders in our minds. Our loads of guilt remain until we allow God to remove them.

The Bible gives us many examples of great men that failed God. How could David become a man after God's own heart when he committed adultery and murder? How could Peter stand and preach to thousands even at the threat of his own death when he'd denied Jesus before a mere maid?

The verse above gives us a four-point answer.

- Admit we did wrong (we were bad).
- Don't be afraid of God's wrath.

From now on, worship God with all your mind, heart and soul. Never turn back to the false gods of food and self-indulgence because they fail.

God's part then kicks in: By His name of truth, He will never abandon you.

Cast off that cloak of guilt. Turn around and start from here.

Prayer: Help me look forward, not at past mistakes.

September 6

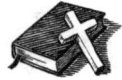

What do I do?

If any of you lack wisdom, let him ask of God, that giveth to all men liberally, and upbraideth not and it shall be given him.
James 1:5

In weight loss classes, I've heard it said, "I just don't know what to do. Nothing has ever worked for me." If this is you, right now, ask God that question. Everything comes from Him. We must have faith to please Him, but even faith comes from Him. Everything begins and ends with God. The Bible calls it "the alpha and omega." We would say that He's everything from A to Z.

So don't think it strange that if you lack wisdom you must ask God for it.

My grandson takes algebra in junior high school. His class is an advanced course and he struggled in the beginning to learn. Both his mother and father are college-educated and his father is a teacher, but they couldn't help. Not surprising, the lessons came in a certain manner from this teacher and only she could answer his "how?" questions.

God made us in a certain manner, and He is the only one with the training manual. Ask Him how to start. Ask Him what plan you should follow, and what foods to eat or leave alone. Each of us was created uniquely, so what works for me might not work for you. Ask Him.

Notice another point in the above verse. He doesn't scold or punish you for asking or for not understanding. Isn't that neat?

Prayer: Lord, show me how to start, what to eat and what
You'd have me do today.

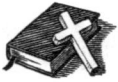

September 7

Grow Deep Roots

Let your roots grow down into him and draw up nourishment from him. See that you go on growing in the Lord, and become strong and vigorous in the truth you were taught. Let your lives overflow with joy and thanksgiving for all he has done.
Colossians 2:7 Life Recovery Bible

In flower pots around our swimming pool, my husband planted zinnias in the spring. During the heat of summer, they wilted, browned, and died. He pulled them up with much of the roots attached. The pot remained empty until now. The weather cooled, and God sent us rain twice. Were we ever surprised to see golden zinnias poking their heads over the edge of the pot! Some roots grew so deep, they resisted the terrible drought and heat. Their strength held until better conditions appeared.

While I went through God's healing, I sent roots into His word searching for more and more strength, better understanding, more vigor. Many times during the last eighteen years have overwhelmed me, but some of my roots were deep enough to hold, so God gave me life again.

Send them deep while you're strong.

Hold on to them when you're weak.

Thank God for them.

Always.

Prayer: Help me grow deeper in You today.

September 8

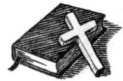

Be a Vigilant Soldier

So be on your guard, not asleep like the others. Watch for his return and stay sober. Night is the time for sleep and the time when people get drunk. But let us who live in the light keep sober, protected by the armor of faith, and love, and wearing as our helmet the happy hope of salvation.
1 Thessalonians 5:6–8. Life Recovery Bible

Darkness brings a time for hidden activities such as drunkenness, sexual impurities, and dwelling on things that divert our attention to what is important. For years, when my husband traveled, I spent my nights worshiping what held my heart. No, I didn't commit adultery with another man, or drink alcohol to knock me out, but I fell before my idol of food. I curled up in my bed with a sack of treats. When sleep claimed me, my body couldn't rest and my mind was clouded with the effects of my sugary sedative.

God desires we be vigilant as a soldier on guard. A soldier who guards the fort or base must remain alert to any enemy. He needs to watch for a change of tactics or a disturbing sound. He must not sleep. He must not drink. His mind should focus on the perils and dangers to his mission.

God uses this comparison to point out how we are to live our renewed lives after receiving His light. We can't ever let down our guard.

Keep on your helmet. Watch and wait. Be sober and alert.

Satan waits at the sideline to seduce us where we're weak and penetrate God's hedge so to entrap us.

Prayer: Lord, guard my mind each moment today.

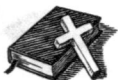

September 9

Keep Me Sensitive

Therefore whosoever heareth these sayings of mine, and doeth them, I will liken him unto a wise man which built upon a rock.
Matthew 7:24

Does anyone besides me remember singing the children's song about the wise man who built his house on the rock and the foolish man who built his on the sand? I love the hand movements that go with the singing especially the *Splat* at the end.

Study this verse. Break it down into sections.

Whoever hears the Word—That's me and you.
So, Jesus is talking directly to us.

Who does what Jesus commands—When we make Jesus Lord of our hearts, we fulfill His command. Again, when we make Him King of our lives, we do His wishes.

That's being wise—Being wise involves doing God's work on earth and that includes being sensitive to others' needs. Jesus exemplified this on earth.

Our house is built on the rock—Our recovery depends on and clings to Jesus.

Have you heard the Word?
Do you do what Jesus asks?
Are you a wise servant?
Do you daily hold to God?

Prayer: Keep me sensitive and wise this day.

September 10

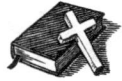

In His Image

And God said Let us make man in our image, after our likeness, and let them have dominion over the fish of the sea, and over the fowl of the air, and over the cattle and over all the earth, and over every creeping thing that creepeth upon the earth. So God created man in his own image, in the image of God created he him, male and female created he them.
Genesis 1:26,27

I view our backyard's flowers, trees and green grass. Birds perch on tree limbs. A cat scampers atop the fence trying to reach the bird's nest. Butterflies kiss trumpet vines. Our neighbor's dog races back and forth on the other side of the fence in an effort to scare the cat.

I think of the first garden created by God, perfect in every way, but there a tiny lamb lay beside a mammoth lion and a snake walked on legs to reach his friend, the hippo. An elephant gave a wasp a free ride. Flowers and trees overflowed with earth's bounty. But God yearned for someone with a free will to adore Him because they chose Him. So He made us.

Just as He told Adam and Eve, He provides thousands of good things, a ton of daily blessings, but He asks only one thing: that we choose to worship Him above everything else and that we commune with Him daily.

God gave us:
- Value
- Capacity to grow
- Availability of His power to overcome anything set on destroying us.

Prayer: I remember today that I was created in Your image, and I seek to honor Your gift.

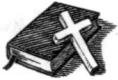

September 11

My Do It Myself

For I the Lord thy God will hold thy right hand, saying unto thee, Fear not; I will help thee. Isaiah 41:13

My oldest daughter and son-in-law bought an inside basketball goal for our first grandchild, their niece. We put it away and brought it out for each one thereafter. By the time, my third and youngest grandchild was born, the basketball goal was worn, but still usable. The pin that held it to a certain height kept getting lost, so I hid it. My grandson loved that goal. By age two, he was wise to my tricks of hiding the pin. He'd drag the whole contraption into the living area and say, "Pin," indicating I should get the lost part. He would take it from my hands and say, "My do it myself."

He would aim and miss several times. I'd say, "Let Mimi do it." But no, "My do it myself." In God-given grandma wisdom, I covered his right hand with mine and guided the pin into the hole. His eyes lit up. Then, he swatted away my hand and reaffirmed, "My do it myself."

What a picture of us at times. We're taught to be independent. When faced with a compulsion we can't control, we argue with ourselves saying, "I'm an accomplished, capable, intelligent woman. I can get on a diet, stay on it and control this thing." But, we try, and try, and can't. No matter how many times we tell God with our actions and words, "my do it myself," we can't.

Finally, God holds our right hand and puts the pieces together. But, too often we still shake His hand away and say, "My do it myself." But we can't. God help us. We never can.

Prayer: When I try to walk in my own power, remind me of my grandson slapping away my hand. God, I need You to hold my right hand.

September 12

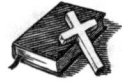

Establish My Work

And let the beauty of the Lord our God be upon us, and establish thou the work of our hands upon us; yes, the work of our hands establish thou it. Psalms 90:17

True success comes from God. Whatever we do daily can bring life, liberty, and prosperity if God initiates it, but it can also bring a valley. Often we pray to ask God's blessing on what we think we need, but prayer should seek God's will, not assume we know it.

Bill W. (Wilson) and Dr. Bob (Smith) began the original Alcoholics Anonymous which has helped thousands of people with alcohol addiction. That beginning spawned others such as Overeaters Anonymous. I've taken part in this group and firmly believe in the teaching.

Prior to 1935, most agree the inspiration for Bill W. and Dr. Bob came in the form of a New York City preacher named Rev. Samuel Moor Shoemaker Jr. of Calvary Episcopal Church. His group of followers became known as the Oxford Group and followed four absolutes: 1) absolute honesty 2) absolute purity 3) absolute love and 4)absolute unselfishness.

Think of applying those absolutes to your work, your gifting or your problem of compulsive overeating. Ask God to establish (create, initiate) the works of your hands. Pray for God's will to be done, not that He bless your will.

Prayer: Let Your beauty be in me, Lord and establish the work of my hands.

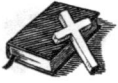

September 13

I Am Strong

Beat your plowshares into swords, and your pruning hooks into spears: let the weak say, I am strong. Joel 3:10

Joel gives us a picture of the end time when Gentile and Jews alike feel beaten and overrun, God tells us to look up because our redemption has come. He advises us to be ready to fight the enemy by using the right tools and encouraging ourselves with the proper words.

Conquering food is easy when everything is going well. We have work to do that interests us, and we're not hungry, tired, lonely, or angry. Our stomachs don't growl. The compulsion doesn't rule. Then, we can confess strength.

Joel describes near the end of the tribulation when nations feel defeated. That's when He reminds us to gather spears and swords and stand in strength—His strength.

Some days I wake up hungry and fight the battle all day. I'm bored, or someone hurt my feelings. I want to clean out the refrigerator and start on the pantry. That's the time when God says to gather our weapons (healthy food, prayer, get up and go—whatever helps you) and claim God's strength. When you're the weakest, that's when God tells us to say: "I am strong."

Are you strong today?

Or, are you strong in Jesus?

Prayer: Remind me today that I am strong regardless of how I feel.

September 14

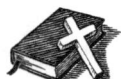

My Life is a Play

Who shall separate us from the love of Christ? Shall tribulation, or distress, or persecution, or famine, or nakedness, or peril, or sword? As it is written, For thy sake we are killed all the day long, we are accounted as sheep for the slaughter. Nay, in all these things we are more than conquerors through him that loved us.
Romans 8: 35-37

I am the director
I place this actor here
And another there
I tell them how to act
And what to say,
Like unruly children
They pay me no mind,
I stamp my feet
And shed my tears
I worry till I am sick
Yet, I must face the fact
I made myself director.
The others take their cues
From God, or from themselves.
I desire, yea demand, perfection,
Yet, I cannot get it
Even from the life God allows me to direct.

By Janet K. Brown

The fate of a compulsive overeater is that of a play's director when the cast, including the leading role, is out of control.

Prayer: Direct my life and everyone in it today.

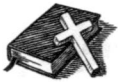

September 15

To Whom Do You Lie?

He that speaketh truth sheweth forth righteousness; but a false witness deceit. Proverbs 12:17

As a Christian, my first answer to the above question would be: "No one. I don't lie." But, that wasn't exactly true. I lied to myself every day.

God created me a special being unique among all humans on earth. How dare I lie to myself and speak bad of His work by calling myself worthless, hopeless or a failure?

Every time I open my mouth to depreciate myself, I lie.

To be **TRUTHful**, I am:
> **T**rustworthy
> **R**ighteous
> **U**seful
> **T**ransformed
> **H**opeful

Through Christ who saves me and molds me into His image.

Prayer: Help me to tell the truth today, even to myself.

September 16

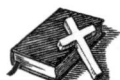

Look in the Mirror

And remember it is a message to obey, not just to listen to. So don't fool yourselves. For if a person just listens and doesn't obey, he is like a man looking at his face in a mirror; As soon as he walks away, he can't see himself anymore or remember what he looks like. James 1: 22-24. Life Recovery Bible

Have you ever passed by a store window and caught a glimpse of your protruding stomach or waddling hips? I don't know about you, but when I saw that, I hastened past, trying to forget. I avoided camera shots because they lay around for years. I couldn't get them out of my mind.

Now, I use those "big" pictures to motivate me and remind me where I came from.

My husband loves store windows. He often stops to comb his hair (a Fonzie want-to-be?). What would we think if he stopped there or at a mirror, looked at his hair, saw a twig standing up on top and never smoothed it down? I would think, "Why bother?"

God wants us to read His word. It's our guidebook for life. His word gives us the steps to navigate our trials and problems. He has the words of life, healing and happiness. Isn't it crazy to look in His word for directions and then turn aside and not smooth off the imperfections we noticed?

Don't *say* you will pray every time you feel tempted to overeat—*do it.*

Don't say you know following God is the only way to victory.

Do ask Him for strength.

Don't just ask wisdom about what to eat.

Buy, prepare, and keep on hand what you know is healthy and good for you.

Prayer: Help me not only look, but help me to DO.

259

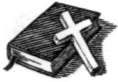

September 17

Give Me a Bigger Foothold

Thou hast enlarged my steps under me that my feet did not slip.
Psalms 18:36

I wish I were creative with my hands. I haven't got a clue how to knit, crochet or sew. I admire people with those skills. Let me tell you about two people who used these skills to solve a problem.

My eighty-eight-year-old mother-in-law lives by herself. All her life she was active and involved. After heart problems and a broken hip confined her to hours of taking life slowly, she experienced loneliness and despair. Taking advantage of her occupation as a seamstress, she turned to quilting to pass the time and make herself feel useful. She's given many family members a Granny quilt. Though her body tires, her attitude blossoms.

A Weight Watcher friend knits potholders to keep her hands busy. Doing this, she lost weight and has maintained the loss for years. She knits two potholders for door prizes to give away at Weight Watcher meetings providing fuel for the old cliché, "killing two birds with one stone."

When we follow God, He weaves our lives into a beautiful creation. Many times we don't like a stitch or a section. We can't see any beauty. But, when years pass and we see the whole design laid out like a path, we often notice He enlarged a place for a foothold when we were in danger of slipping off course. I thank God for helping me past the danger points and following His plan and not mine.

Prayer: Enlarge my steps so that I won't slip.

September 18

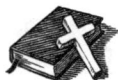

Seal My Lips

Help me, Lord, to keep my mouth shut and my lips sealed.
Psalms 141:3 Life Recovery Bible

This verse speaks to me today. Sometimes, I think the more I talk about God or praise Him with my lips, the holier I will appear. But, our unruly mouths more often get us into trouble.

Our mouths open to take in unneeded extra food.

Our mouths open to speak against others.

Gossip and harsh words fill our mouths.

How can we listen for the needs of others when we talk all the time?

But, what about saying praise to God?

Not a bad thing. But,

It is our lives not our lips that truly praise God.

Death to self helps our prayer life. When we devote ourselves to hear from God, we shut our mouths even in prayer. No longer desirous of laying our petitions before God, we become willing to listen to what He has to say to us.

When temptation rears its ugly head, we need to fall to our knees, seal our lips, and allow God to defend and protect.

The more I think about it, the more I cling to that verse.

Prayer: Lord, keep my mouth shut and my lips sealed today.

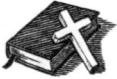

September 19

I Was Destroying Myself

O, Israel, thou hast destroyed thyself; but in me is thine help.
Hosea 13:9

God speaks plainly here to His people. I think He would say the same thing to anyone beset with an addiction or compulsion. A couple of verses down, He tells Israel that He gave them a king in His anger and then took away the king at His pleasure. A Christian life isn't run by democracy. God is sovereign. If we place something or someone else as king of our lives, He might allow it in His anger knowing that it will destroy us.

God created us to serve Him. Only He can fill that special place in our spirit created for communion with God. Any substitute is destructive. Anything else on the throne ruins us. Another king prevents God's wonderful plans from coming to pass.

Compulsive overeating = Destruction

God = A thing of beauty

For years, I yearned for happiness, but dissolved into despair. I would ask God to take away my craving for sweets and my huge appetite.

Now I see how my request resembled one given by a six-year-old and posted online. "I'm thankful for this baby brother, but what I really wanted was a puppy."

I asked God for happiness and control of my eating, but what I really wanted was to eat like I wanted and be thin.

When I finally gave in to His control, He gave me Himself and that brought me appetite control with true happiness.

Prayer: What I want today is for God to be king.

September 20

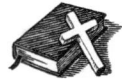

I'm Helpless

I am the vine, ye are the branches. He that abideth in me, and I in him, the same bringeth forth much fruit: for without me ye can do nothing. John 15:5

My husband occasionally cuts off the stems from his rose bushes to make a lovely rose bouquet. At first, the arrangement is gorgeous and blesses our entire house with beauty and a delightful fragrance.

Gradually, petals drop, leaves turn brown and the smell isn't so good. Within ten days to two weeks, all the blossoms are gone, and even the stem withers and dies.

What's the difference? The roses outside are still a lush green. New blossoms replace the dying ones. But, in my bouquet, death wins out. The difference is the outside flowers remain in the vine.

When we isolate ourselves from communion with God, we receive no nourishment. Death stalks us and will ultimately win. The Word says it best: without Christ, we can do nothing. In Christ, we are beautiful, our fragrance wafts through our family and touches our friends, because we have life.

Christ came to give us life—life to be what He wants us to be. Wait for the life-giving nourishment from the vine before you attempt any challenge. That includes a new way of eating.

Prayer: I'll remain in God as a branch stays in the vine.

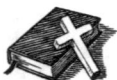

September 21

Victory from Overeating

When an evil spirit comes out of a man, it goes through arid places seeking rest and does not find it. Then, it says, I will return to the house I left. When it arrives, it finds the house swept clean and put in order. Then, it goes and takes seven other spirits more wicked than itself, and they go in and live there. And the final condition of that man is worse than the fist. Luke 11:24-26 NIV

Through years of eating, bingeing, and eating again, I conquered my craving for food many times. When I proclaimed victory from overeating, I felt powerful, just, triumphant. But over time, my weight crept up again, my spirits sagged.

God gave me the problem of food addiction to draw me to ask for His help. When I felt justified and perfect, I didn't need God. But, when I failed, I did. God wants us to seek Him with a passion. Sometimes, even when we seek His help and allow Him to guide us in this problem, our motivation is to lose weight. Weight loss is a good thing, but God craves our devotion. Our reason for seeking Him should be to draw close to God, to have more of Him in our life.

When we rid ourselves of compulsive eating and the sins of anger and resentments, we are like the man swept clean of evil. Our house is set in order, the heavy spirit of wickedness is gone, leaving a void in our lives. Fill up your house with Jesus. When you give your heart to Him, He puts into you a new spirit. Let that new spirit fill your life. Seek to read the Word more, to pray, praise, and seek His face. Fill your house with God.

Jesus warns us. When we clean our lives of evil, it seeks to return. When this happens, we are worse than before. How many times have I lost fifty pounds, only to fail and put sixty back in its place? Read the verses above and learn.

Prayer: Fill my life to overflowing.

September 22

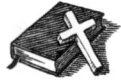

Are You Thirsty?

In the last day, that great day of the feast, Jesus stood and cried saying, 'If any man thirst, let him come unto me and drink'.
John 7:37

My husband and I love the mountains. Streams cut a path through the peaks, so often the highways follow the stream's natural winding. Once, we parked and walked beside the river. I was so thirsty, but we had drunk the last water in our cooler, and it would take half hour to reach the next town to buy more.

The bubbling brook mocked my thirst, enticing me with what I craved. I lay on a rock and attempted to scoop water with my hands, but I dribbled more than I got down my throat.

Charles remembered he had a Styrofoam cup half-filled with cola. "You can have this," he said. I didn't want a cola. My doctor had told me to avoid them. I wanted water.

"Then pour out the cola," Charles said.

I returned to the car, took the cup and poured it out on the ground. Now, my cup was empty of what harmed me. I leaned over a rock, filled up the cup with life-giving water and drank my fill. (I realize we're warned to not drink from streams except when worried about dehydration. This is for example purposes only.)

What if I'd held onto that cup and prayed, "God, I've gotten rid of the offensive thing in my cup. It's empty now. Please fill it with water?" I think I hear the Lord laughing and thinking that He already provided the water. It was right in front of me, looking delicious and wholesome. All I needed to do was fill it.

Friend, if that's you who has emptied your body of over-eating, look to God. He's provided the water of life to fill your body, your mind and your soul. Are you thirsty?

Prayer: Open my eyes how to fill my vessel with You.

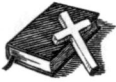

September 23

Prepare Against Surfeiting

And take heed to yourselves, lest at any time your hearts be overcharged with surfeiting, and drunkenness, and cares of this life, and so that day come upon you unawares. Luke 21:34

The King James version of the Bible uses old English words that we don't use today, but I want to look at the meaning of the words in this verse. My Bible gives this passage in red letters to inform us that they're Jesus' own words while He was here on earth.

Jesus warns us of:
1. Surfeiting
2. Drunkenness
3. Cares of this life

I understand drunkenness. Recovering alcoholics must particularly guard against this temptation. Party times become a problem. Alcoholics must be careful.

Cares of this life can catch any of us. If activities, even good ones, keep us from worshipping and spending time with God, that thing becomes a snare.

Jesus aims the word surfeiting to people like me. Surfeiting means overindulging, gorging, stuffing even to the point that the word is used for discomfort or nausea. We try to apply this only to people who are overweight, but this applies to everyone. If we've ever backed away from the table uncomfortable because of overindulgence, we are guilty. When we think more about our taste buds than we think about God, food snares us.

Beware of surfeiting, drunkenness and cares of this life. Americans, in the land of excess, suffer from all three maladies.

Prayer: Lord, keep me watchful for these sneaky sins.

September 24

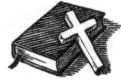

Children Lead

Whomsoever therefore shall humble himself as this little child, the same is greatest in the kingdom of heaven. Matthew 18:4

Children are open books. They have no intimidation and no fear that they'll say or do the wrong thing. They speak what they think while a people-pleaser like me worries over everything I did or didn't do. True, children embarrass their parents and grandparents at times, but how often we wish we could be that carefree.

This evening I watched my music minister's seven-year-old son direct his own "choir" from his front row seat. On the platform, his dad swung his arms in tempo to the music. The son did the same without concern who might be watching. He merely imitated his dad, knowing there would be no harm in doing so.

While on earth, Jesus consulted His father every day, asking guidance for every decision, every thought, every action. He didn't seek insight from his peers, friend or foe, but only God's direction. Our friends may try a new diet or join a new gym, but our direction must come from heaven. Like my music minister's young son, we must not consider others' decisions, only God's. Follow Him in lock step with humility and the openness of a child.

Have you watched a child lately? Whom does he wish to impress? Probably, his mother or father, or maybe a favorite teacher. With an open heart, he does what that person likes. Ask God to Help you to do what God desires.

Prayer: Give me the humility and open heart of a child.

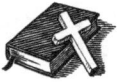

September 25

Clean The Inside

Woe unto you scribes and Pharisees, hypocrites, for ye make clean the outside of the cup and of the platter, but within they are full of extortion and excess. Matthew 23:25

When my youngest daughter reached five, she loved to help in the kitchen. She liked cooking best of all, but she even helped with dish-washing, preferring to act big, like her Momma. I scrambled eggs and stuck them to the bottom of my skillet. My daughter dropped the pan in sudsy water and rubbed it with a dishrag. She laid it aside to dry.

I picked up the skillet. "This isn't clean," I told her.

Did she not see the egg coating? I pushed her out of the way, took my scrubber and cleaned the skillet.

She smiled sweetly. "But, I did a good job on the outside, didn't I, Mommy?"

Since she was a child, I could love her just for trying so hard, but when we reach adulthood, the outside isn't enough. Jesus called religious leaders of the day "hypocrites" and claimed they only cleaned the outside, while the inside was filthy.

Eating limited calories or refraining from eating desserts may seem wholesome and desirable, but that's only cleaning the outside if your heart still dwells on what you missed.

If two women eat lunch and one has salad and the other has cheesecake, we judge the salad lady as righteous. Indeed, she might be, but just eating the salad with no dressing doesn't make her sinless with her eating. Bowing before God that morning and repenting of repeated thoughts about food is what makes her whole. At the same time, the dessert eater might bow her head and thank God for allowing her a sweet taste of cheesecake, and go away justified.

Prayer: Make me whole, Lord, inside and out.

September 26

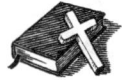

Did I Do Enough?

For John came neither eating nor drinking, and they say, He hath a devil. The Son of man came eating and drinking, and they say Behold a man gluttonous, and a winebibber, a friend of publicans and sinners. But wisdom is justified of her children.
Matthew 11:18,19

Jesus told of how people compared the actions of John the Baptist and himself while on earth. People today are quick to judge what or how we eat too, especially if we're overweight.

My mother berated me for being fat but then was hurt when I didn't indulge in special pies or treats that she prepared. People can be two-faced hypocrites, as Jesus called the Pharisees. I'll admit that I'm the worst of them all, but we should guard against a critical attitude.

After our Christian Weight Controller group at church stopped, I joined a Weight Watcher meeting to finish losing my weight. The plan wasn't that much different than the American Diabetic exchange diet I followed. I'm an organized, regimented person, so I preferred a guideline of healthy eating.

Other people have lost weight by leaving off certain foods or watching portions. So as not to get hungry, many eat several meals a day such as the "Flat Belly" diet admonishes. With me, eating between meals was a hindrance, so I stuck with three complete meals and one light, planned snack.

I have good, well-meaning Weight Watcher friends that journal and attend meetings every week even after reaching goals. That works for them. I've known many who exercise constantly and some who never do. There is no wrong way. But it is wrong to criticize others for not doing what you do. God has a plan for each of us to follow. That's always enough.

Prayer: Lord, keep my eating on the right track for You.

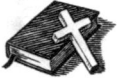

September 27

My Glory

And to all who received him, he gave the right to become children of God. All they needed to do was to trust him to save them.
John 1:12 Life Recovery Bible

Everything we do prepares us for His glory.
How we eat.
How we talk.
How we act.
How we relate to others.
Our attitude.
Our critical manner.
How much we yearn for His Word.
How we do the work of our lives.

God plans our lives before we're born. He attempts to transform us so we might enter into His glory. If we allow it, He will change our destinies, not just our behavior.

Think about it. If He can change the way we look at food, He can transform the plans for our lives and the glory that awaits us in heaven. All because we turned over our food to Him.

Prayer: Take my food, my choices, my will today. Transform me into Your glory.

September 28

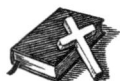

Move Me Out of the Way

One of the two which heard John speak, and followed him was Andrew, Simon Peter's brother. He first findeth his own brother Simon, and saith unto him, we have found the Messias, which is, being interpreted, the Christ. John 1:40,41

Our church is having revival services this week. Already, the devil is fighting me with my old foes—resentment and envy. Last night, I prayed around the altar. I asked God to speak through me, but always someone else moved in to the petitioner and out-prayed me. People turned to other people, not me. I left feeling rejected and useless.

This morning, God sent me to the above Scripture first thing. We learn little of Andrew in the Scripture, but in these verses, Andrew first follows Christ and tells his brother about Him. From then on, Andrew takes a back seat. Jesus chooses Peter as one of the three closest to Him. It's Peter that witnesses the transfiguration, not his brother. It's Peter that Jesus asks to pray for Him in the garden, not Andrew. And it's Peter that preaches the first sermon after Pentecost.

Andrew waited in the background but was faithful. God desired to highlight the above action of Andrew in His Word as an example to ones like me who don't get recognition.

The Bible tells of others, such as Barnabas, who stayed in the shadows and let Paul shine. Naomi grew older, stepped back, and let Ruth take the forefront. God shows different servants to remind us of how we all fit together in the kingdom.

I prayed that God would stop the resentment and envy troubling my spirit because if those thoughts remain, I will overeat and sin against God's healing. Today's verse helped me.

Prayer: Lord, keep my mind fixed on You so that I might follow Your plan for my life.

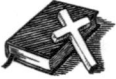

September 29

Prepare for the Unexpected

to prepare God's people for works of service, so that the body of Christ may be built up until we all reach unity in the faith and to the knowledge of the Son of God and become mature, attaining to the whole measure of the fullness of Christ. Ephesians 4:13 NIV

This verse encourages us to prepare for perfection though we never attain that ideal in this life. That's true also of our weight recovery.

Always prepare for the unexpected.

Watch out for temptation's snare.

Anticipate problem areas.

Lay the groundwork for victory by visiting with the Lord early in your day.

Arrange your food supply to include easy and healthy options.

Visualize what you'll do at a party or celebration.

Allow time to encourage others.

The verse following the one above tells where we start and why we prepare.

Then we will no longer be infants, tossed back and forth by the waves, and blown here and there by every wind of teaching, and by the cunning and craftiness of men in their deceitful scheming. Ephesians 4:14 NIV

In the throes of my food compulsion, the tossing waves influenced my life. After God healed me, I began to prepare for perfection.

Prayer: Lord, help me to further groom my life for Your ideal.

September 30

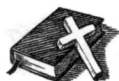

Broken

The Lord is nigh unto them that are of a broken heart; and saveth such as be of a contrite spirit. Psalms 34:18

In 1993, I came to God, a broken individual, no longer able to cope with life. Like a broken toy, I felt cast aside, dysfunctional, and miserable. I no longer wanted to live. I saw little hope for my future. I told God that if He could do anything for me, to start now, because I was through trying.

At that point, I could not envision that my circumstances were what God had been waiting for. My pastor recently preached on the subject of brokenness. He told us, "God uses broken people, not confident, strong people." How true.

Strong, confident individuals work too hard. They prefer independence, control and self-directed purpose. For God to mold us according to His purpose, that streak of I-can-do-it-myself must be dashed, trampled and vanquished.

Then, He rebuilds us.

Have you ever watched a child play? My grandson diligently builds a fort with his Legos, then kicks the pieces, scattering them here and yon, because He wants to improve it. The next time he builds it, his masterpiece improves.

God uses broken people. We must remain pliable and usable in His hands. With brokenness, His masterpiece only improves.

Prayer: Do with me today as You would.

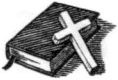

October 1

Symptom of a Spiritual Lapse

Now learn a parable of the fig tree, When his branch is yet tender and putteth forth leaves, ye know that summer is nigh. So likewise ye when ye shall see all these things, know that it is near, even at the doors. Matthew 24: 32,33

Jesus uses nature to explain things in terms we humans can understand. In chapter 24 of Matthew, Jesus' own words gave signs of the end of the age. In the above verses, He explains that we can see these signs and know what's coming. We know better how to pray.

When Israel won its independence and once again became a country, the people in that generation realized they should pray, "Yea, Lord, come quickly." Today, with the increase in weather turbulence, wars and earthquakes, we realize our time is short to work for God.

When a Christmas cactus stretches out fragile shoots at the end of each stem, we know blooms are coming. When tree leaves turn red or gold, we know they soon will fall. When our physical bodies give us pain, chills, or high temperature as symptoms, we know to seek help.

When rebellion builds in our minds and we want more food or different foods, we realize that's a symptom that we're in trouble spiritually. Fall on your knees. Ask the heavenly physician to highlight what's wrong. Focus on Him. It's all about God. His x-ray images point out the trouble areas—not enough prayer, getting too busy, letting our thoughts dwell too much on ourselves.

When we allow God to diagnose our problem and fix it, we no longer want extra food. God uses our desire to overeat as a sign of how to pray.

Prayer: When symptoms arise, help me run to Doctor Jesus.

October 2

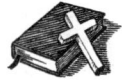

Good, Better, Best

And Jesus answered and said unto her, Martha, Martha, thou art careful and troubled about many things. But one thing is needful and Mary hath chosen that good part, which shall not be taken away from her. Luke 10:41-42

I have a friend who works so hard for God. She uses up her body helping the widows, the elderly, and the sick. She pushes herself to take part in three or four Bible studies at a time, usually teaching at least one of them. She picks up trash along the highway near her, races for the cure for breast cancer and sells books at the library to raise money to keep it open. She's a busy person. Like Martha in Jesus' story from the verses above, my friend chooses the good.

Martha was a friend to Jesus. She desired everything to be perfect for Him because she loved Him. But, because she stewed over that perfection, she missed an opportunity to relax and sit in His presence. Her sister, on the other hand, failed to help out and take some of the load off Martha. Yet, Jesus explains that Mary selected the best.

Good—Better—Best

Jesus says the best part is sitting in His presence and listening to Him. How long has it been since you've done that?

Yes, there's a time for service. Our love for God spurs us to help others, to donate time and money, to teach, to learn, but we must be careful that those times never push out "the best part."

More than any other group, overeaters and other addicted or compulsive individuals need to stop, relax and listen.

Prayer: Speak to me today, Lord. I'm waiting and listening.

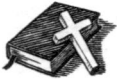

October 3

Who's in the Driver's Seat?

Ye have sown much and bring in little; ye eat, but ye have not enough, ye drink, but ye are not filed with drink, ye clothe you, but there is none warm, and he that earneth wages earneth wages to put it into a bag with holes. Haggai 1:6

When God's people returned from exile, they began to rebuild the temple of God, but the devil sidetracked them with selfish desires. They stopped work on God's temple and built their own homes. Their time went into their own crops and orchards and harvesting and putting away for themselves. Oh, they still went through the form of worshipping God, but their lives revealed who was most important to them.

My mother had many sayings. One of the few I understood stands out: "put it on the back burner." In the days before microwaves, the cook kept soup, tea or something else on a low flame at the back of the stove. She cooked the immediate meal at the front. That was what she planned on serving, but the back burner held something that she kept warm in case someone wanted it. Back burner items were incidental. To the Israelites in the verse above, God became incidental.

God spoke to them to examine their lives. Though they worked hard to satisfy their needs, it was never enough.

How many of us eat one thing and then another, seeking just the right flavor, but are never satisfied? We, like the Israelites above, should examine our lives. Are we content? Is God in the driver's seat? Are we pushing ourselves to exhaustion in a life that can never bring peace or fulfillment?

Is God in the driver's seat, or do you keep Him in the back seat while you drive?

Prayer: Take over my life, today, Lord. You, drive.

October 4

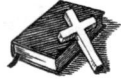

Confounded or Consumed?

For the Lord God will help me; therefore shall I not be confounded; therefore have I set my face like a flint, and I know that I shall not be ashamed. Isaiah 50:7

All this new technology confuses me. Just about the time I think I have blogging or Facebook figured out, it messes up, and I'm overwhelmed with learning to fix it. I'm a simple person. I resist change. Since the computer isn't something I like, I want to quit. But, when I decide to do something that matters to me, I refuse to give up on it.

I love the way I feel without the burden of ninety-five extra pounds on my body. My energy level has doubled. My health is better than thirty years ago. I don't mind shopping since I can look for regular-sized clothes and not oversized. In the past, shopping brought depression because nothing fit. Weight loss and now weight maintenance is important to me.

God's way of weight loss is simple.
Ask Him in the morning what to eat.
Concentrate on Him and not yourself.
Set your face toward His Word (like a flint).
Be proud of who you are in Christ. (Don't be ashamed.)
Rely on God's power, not your weak will, so you won't be
    confounded or dismayed.

Prayer: Help. I'm stuck again.

277

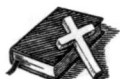

October 5

Obedience

Know ye not that to whom ye yield yourselves servants to obey, his servants ye are to whom ye obey; whether of sin unto death or of obedience unto righteousness. Romans 6:16

What rules your life?
Whom do you turn in the fray?
Who is it you love?
It's who you obey.

Jesus said that if we love Him, we will obey Him.

You'll serve someone
No matter life's station
If you turn away from God,
You become slave to Satan.

There's a song "You're Gonna Serve Someone." It points out that, regardless of your station in life, either you will serve God or you will serve Satan by default.

Jesus told us we can't serve mammon and God. If we hold onto God, we drop our idols. If we cling to an idol (food), we quit serving God.

Examine your life.
Whom do you love?
If you say Jesus,
 He'll be enough.

Prayer: Remind me of what true love to Christ means—
obedience.

October 6

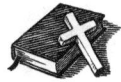

What's the Best Tool?

(For the weapons of our warfare are not carnal but mighty through God to the pulling down of strongholds.)
2 Corinthians 10:4

A soldier chooses the correct weapon to fight. Sometimes, that might be a small gun, but other times, they require a tank or grenade. A house builder picks the right size drill or a particular kind of screwdriver.

When we turn our lives over to Jesus, we enlist in a spiritual war. The devil is our enemy and seeks to destroy. He doesn't fight fair. He looks at our weaknesses and hits us in those areas.

For a compulsive overeater or one prone to emotional upheaval, Satan strikes with the temptations that debilitated us in the past. Choose the correct tool to fight him.

"If the only tool you have is a hammer, you tend to see every problem as a nail." Abraham Maslow

When we react quickly without prayer, without planning, we use a hammer when sandpaper might work best. When a neighbor comes over with a pan of fudge, don't panic and think "I must eat it if she thought enough of me to cook them." That's "using a nail" philosophy. Instead, take it slow and steady like rubbing sandpaper over a rough edge.

Step back.
Be grateful.
Detach from the immediate weakness.
Pray
Eat an apple or a meal if it's time
Use the proper tools to battle.

Prayer: Help me take a breath and wait for Your guidance.

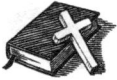

October 7

Twisted and Tied

And I will be found of you, saith the Lord; and I will turn away your captivity, and I will gather you from all the nations, and from all the places whither I have driven you, saith the Lord, and I will bring you again into the place whence I caused you to be carried away captive. Jeremiah 29:14

Ask my husband. It's impossible for me to lie still when I sleep. I toss from my stomach to my left side, from my right side to my back and over then again. I can't wear a long gown or pajama bottoms. They tie me in knots. Once, on a very cold night, I wore a full length flannel gown. In the morning, I awoke like a mummy, bound to the point I couldn't move. My husband had to unravel the tangle before I could climb from bed.

That was funny, but food tied and tangled me in the same manner, and that wasn't amusing. God stood by and watched while I twisted until food captured my life and held me prisoner to the demands of overeating. My emotions bound me in a tight cell and allowed for little joy or coping ability.

Just as with the people of Israel, God promises that if we call on Him, He will release us from captivity and bring us back to the place of happiness and freedom.

Has self pity and your love of food twisted and tied you in knots where you need help to function? It took my husband's strength to unbind me from a tangled gown. Only the power of God can release us from the captivity of compulsion.

Prayer: Deliver me from food's imprisonment.

October 8

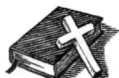

The Lord is My Shepherd
Psalm 23

Sleepless nights plague me when I have a lot on my mind or I'm not feeling well. Often, I turn to the twenty-third Psalm. God gave these words to David, I believe, to settle believers' minds and bodies. Recently, God again brought the words to my thoughts with an interpretation that I needed for that moment.

Verse 1—The Lord is my shepherd; I shall not want.

Nothing catches my Lord by surprise. He stands beside my bed with weapon drawn to protect me from any enemy the devil sends my way. When I need healing, He provides; when peace, he supplies; when it's help for my family, He summons angels to get to work. He's my shepherd, my protector, my provider, my healer, my all in all. I never want.

Verse 2—*He maketh me to lie down in green pastures; he leadeth me beside still waters.*

Green pastures summon a picture of rural, simple, peaceful valleys away from the hustle of computers, phones, and argumentative people. God leads us to that place where we're shut away from fast-paced, hectic, urban jumble. There, His voice speaks to us, and we can hear.

When my husband and I were young parents, we drove to a nearby lake and watched the water slowly ripple to the land. Beside still water, we find truth and direction for our lives. God created that in us and provides it when we ask.

In Jack Canfield's *The Success Principles,* he suggests that when we go to bed, the last thing on our minds should be our goal. While we sleep, our subconscious works on ways to reach the destination we desire.

Prayer: Tonight, when I go to bed, set my thoughts on the twenty-third Psalm.

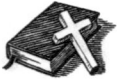

October 9

The Valley of the Shadow of Death
Psalm 23

Verse 3—He restoreth my soul; he leadeth me in the paths of righteousness for his name's sake.

The pace of our busy lives gives us a rough edge. We become cynical, angry and full of doubt. God likens that to losing our soul. The world destroys our God-given, child-like innocence. In that green pasture and beside those still waters, He restores that to us. God imparts His righteousness, His glory, His truth and rebuilds our ability to believe, to trust as our children once trusted us.

Verse 4—Yea, though I walk through the valley of the shadow of death, I will fear no evil, for thou art with me; thy rod and thy staff they comfort me.

Again, we see the picture of the good shepherd as Jesus described himself in the book of John. The rod and staff signify the appropriate weapons to conquer our problems.

The valley of the shadow of death reminds us that death and all personal trials come to us alone, away from loved ones and friends. Of course, we cherish and long for their comfort, but when I battle resentment and hurt feelings, when I want to buy a dozen donuts and eat them all, I'm alone in that war. Only God can travel with me. But He will not insist. We must invite Him. Don't forget to ask for His presence first, regardless of the turmoil.

Prayer: Never cease to walk and protect me. I know not what lies ahead today.

October 10

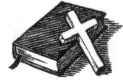

Goodness and Mercy Required
Psalm 23

Verse 5—Thou preparest a table before me in the presence of mine enemies: thou anointest my head with oil; my cup runneth over.

Before God created Adam and Eve, He brought forth fruits and grains for food. Food to man has always been a source of celebration and enjoyment. Compulsive overeaters tend to classify foods as good or bad. Lettuce is good. Cheesecake is bad. Yet God provides all foods and combinations thereof that man has developed for our pleasure. God is a giver. He prepares a table of food to give us joy. Food and fellowship go together. Even when enemies (temptations, anger) abound, He provides a good table and is willing to guide our choices. Food isn't bad. Overindulgence is what sacrifices our peace.

The word anoint comes from a Latin word meaning "spread with oil" and is used one hundred fifty times in the Bible. Oil can be medicinal (soothing, healing), aromatic (sense of well being, charismatic), and ritualistic (meaning to set apart for the Holy Spirit, to consecrate, free and prepare.) In the Old Testament, the oil represented the presence of God.

Verse 6—Surely goodness and mercy shall follow me all the days of my life; and I will dwell in the house of the Lord for ever.

Somehow, after that verse, I wish to merely say "Amen." Fill my cup to overflowing with goodness and mercy now and hope for the future with God.

Prayer: I need Your goodness, mercy and celebration of food daily, according to Your direction.

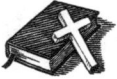

October 11

God in the Storm

But soon a terrible storm arose. High waves began to break into the boat until it was nearly full of water and about to sink.
Jesus was asleep at the back of the boat with his head on a cushion. Frantically, they wakened him, shouting, 'Teacher, don't you even care that we are all about to drown?'
Mark 4:35,36 Live Recovery Bible

During the storm, we stew and worry. We tremble and cringe. We see no escape. Jesus appears to be asleep in the back of the boat, oblivious to our plight. The last week, I've been in the storm. Rain blinded my trust-ability. Blustery winds concealed the sound of His voice. Two days ago, I "hit the wall." Exhaustion, illness, worry and my usual struggle with resentment took a toll on my mind and my body. I sought to "wake up" my Lord. With tears streaming my face, I cried out, "Don't you care that I perish?"

God answered me as he did the disciples long ago. He spoke to the storm: "Quiet down." The wind and rain diminished. Then, He turned to me and asked why I was so fearful. "Didn't you know I was with you?"

Recently, I saw an anonymous saying that I thought God would have me remember.

Life isn't about waiting for the storm to pass. It's learning how to dance in the rain.

Prayer: Lord, even while the storm rages, teach me to dance.

October 12

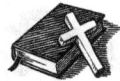

Excuses

Then we went to the Fountain Gate and to the King's Pool; but my donkey couldn't get through the rubble. So we circled the city and I followed the brook, inspecting the wall, and entered again at the Valley Gate. Nehemiah 2: 14,15 Life Recovery Bible

Salvation doesn't immediately show us all our faults. Salvation turns us to the right path to God. To keep us from stumbling, His flashlight points out the dips and holes on the road. So, too, in our journey of emotional healing, we mustn't expect perfection. Periodic inspections reveal areas we can improve or detours we should take.

God gave Nehemiah the task of rebuilding the wall of Israel. After getting the okay of the king, Nehemiah returned to his homeland. At first look, he determined he couldn't even get through the rubble to see the wall, but undeterred, he found another way. The job took years and trials on end, but this man of God fulfilled his destiny.

So, too, we can finish the task God has given to compulsive overeaters.

After we start off, we should, from time to time, submit to God in new areas when He reveals them to us. Some of the cracks or breaks in the wall escaped Nehemiah's notice on the first inspection or the second or third, but he kept rechecking. No excuses. This is a journey of growth.

Excuses are the disintegrating blacktop on the road or the rotten wood of the bridge. Replace them with new material and wonder at its strength.

Prayer: Take away my excuse. Reveal new areas I need to open to the light.

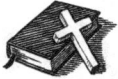

October 13

What's My Problem?

There is a way that seemeth right unto man; but the end thereof are the ways of death. Proverbs 16:25

For four years, my daughter's family has struggled with job insecurity, put-downs from neighbors, rush-rush turmoil of a life out of control and no relief when they pray. As this last year neared closure, they examined their lives. Where had they gone wrong? Yes, the younger boy grew older and became more involved in his own activities. True, my daughter's drive from work to home had tripled. But, the family was strong. Their children were happy. They loved a full life. The difference came in the time before God. Unlike their schedule before their last move, the busyness had choked out church. They got plenty of good stuff, but not always God's stuff.

My Bible warns me that often what I think is the right thing to do isn't. Not if I act according to my own wisdom. That wisdom is human and faulty even though I see it as good and proper. My daughter could see the love in her family, the strength of her marriage, the reasons for what they did and believed she traveled the correct path for her life. Our way seems *right to us*, but only God's way leads to life.

But seek ye first his kingdom and his righteousness and all these things will be give to you as well. Matthew 6:33 NIV

This verse reminds us to seek God first. Only then will each part of our lives fall into place, not without problems, but always for our good.

Prayer: Today, I seek Your counsel first.

October 14

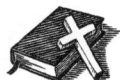

Abandon

Wherefore, my beloved, as ye have always obeyed, not as in my presence only, but now much more in my absence, work out your own salvation with fear and trembling. Philippians 2:12

Inch by inch, step by step, we work out our salvation along with God. No one else can walk the path with us. Each person's plan differs. What seems foolish to one, brings life to another. At a crossroad, we look to God. He shows light to one area of our lives and then another. Regardless of whether you just turned your life over to His control today or forty years ago, we are beginners. God's path is exciting. We never know what lies ahead, but we know who leads as we abandon one area after another and leave it to His control.

Abandon:
A ll of me
B roach a change of direction
A dopt a God perspective
N o matter how it looks to me
D iscard old habits
O pen to His voice
N ovice

Prayer: As a novice, I abandon what I know of life and follow You.

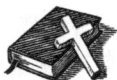

October 15

Lose That Burden

And now, through Christ, all the kindness of God has been poured out upon us undeserving sinners, and now he is sending us out around the world to tell all people everywhere the great things God has done for them, so that they, too, will believe and obey him. And you, dear friends in Rome, are among those he dearly loves; you, too, are invited by Jesus Christ to be God's very own— yes, his holy people. Romans 1:5,6 Life Recovery Bible

When I lost the weight from my physical body, I found I still lugged the burden on my mind. Do you find that true? I'm here to say, "throw out that burden."

Paul's mission to the Gentiles was one of hope. Jews were God's holy nation. He gave them His law and from their loins came the Messiah. Gentiles could never hope to catch up with the Jews in learning all the rules. Because of this, Israelites looked down on anyone else in the world as hopeless to please God. But, God sent out Paul to preach the good tidings to the Gentiles. God now included them as His children. He poured out blessings on the Greeks and even the Romans. They, too could become the children of God. What good news!

Liberty from overeating isn't reserved for the few. God provides it to anyone willing to let go, anyone who submits the problem to Him.

My choices for food or activity aren't listed as right or wrong, but merely as good for me or not a wise choice. When I indulge in two pieces of cake, I'm not bad. I chose unwisely. Next time, remember what didn't work. Rigid eating plans tie us in knots. God gives freedom, hope and joy. Keep reading further in the book.

Prayer: Take away my need for unyielding laws and give me liberty.

October 16

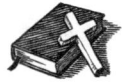

I'm Not the Master of Anything

Brethren, I count not myself to have apprehended; but this one thing I do, forgetting those things which are behind, and reaching forth unto those things which are before. I press toward the mark for the prize of the high calling of God in Christ Jesus.
Philippians 3:13,14

The need for perfection riddled my life with imperfection.

Today, I admit I haven't mastered this walk, nor will I ever, this side of heaven. Don't think I'm the expert in this area. I'm learning and walking this path same as you, my friend. With every devotion I write, I read because I need it. Sometimes I think God gave me these devotions just for my benefit.

Under God's inspiration, Paul wrote many letters. Yet, in the verses above, he reminds us that he hasn't yet attained the goal. You and I must read his advice and apply it to our lives.

Forget the things that have gone before.

- The diet plans tried and failed.
- The times we didn't turn to God and overate.
- The trips to the altar to "let go" when we picked up the vice again and took it home with us.

Reach forth to those things to come. Walk one step at a time but have hope for the future.

Why? Because we have faith in God, the author and finisher of hope.

I press on. I persevere.

When I falter, I pick myself up, look for God's flashlight and push forward.

The prize of heaven dazzles Christians, but a prize right now is a God-controlled eating plan. The prize now is good health, more energy, quality of life, and perhaps easier later years.

Prayer: I follow Jesus, the Master.

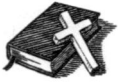

October 17

Look Up

I will lift up mine eyes unto the hills, from whence cometh my help. Psalms 121:1

Some will read this devotion only to be burdened with more humiliation and self loathing because, so far, you haven't obtained Christ's freedom in the area of weight recovery. I bear good news.

God is never late. His mercies are new every day and available when you're open to acceptance. Most compulsive overeaters reach their bottom when they've tried every diet plan imaginable. (Like me). Each bottom differs from someone else's lowest point. When we drop to our lowest, we give up. Only then can God work.

God looks on when we gorge on cheesecake or stuff our mouths with chocolate. God watches when we lay with upset stomach and pounding headache after a binge. He waits for us. When we can't stand ourselves any longer, He's there to pick up the pieces. When we reach the point of total depravity in our own eyes, we can accept His power. Praise God. Look up. Your redemption draws nigh.

"Those times of self-humiliation are the most unlovely and unwelcome hours of the Christian life; but they grow power and joy and peace, as rotten earth grows roses." Rev. Sam Shoemaker's sermon in *Courage to Change* by Bill Pittman and Dick B.

Prayer: Thank You, Lord, for standing ready to catch me when I fall.

October 18

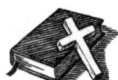

Self Control

It is better to be slow-tempered than famous; it is better to self-control than to control an army.
Proverbs 16:32 Life Recovery Bible

When I lose my temper, I'm embarrassed. I learned instead to bite my tongue so everyone thought I was sweet and calm-mannered, then I would binge eat. The anger remained but turned inward. Anger at my actions lowered my view of myself which further isolated me from people. I thought others wouldn't like me if they knew the real me.

I hate talking about self-control. The thought makes me nervous. I'd rather be famous. But, God tells me in Proverbs, that's not the best. Like you, I'd like to be self controlled, but I know I fall short of the goal. Something about the term sounds like I have to do it by myself. Then, why did the Bible list it as a fruit of the Spirit?

S elfish	**S** avior
E ating our feelings	**P** atience
L ow self-esteem	**I** llumination
F ailure	**R** ighteousness of God
	I ncredible power
	T emperance

I choose to believe the word self-control is an oxymoron. Self control isn't from self at all. Only the Holy Spirit offers the fruit of self-control.

Prayer: Lord, give me Spirit-control today and forever.

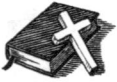

October 19

Pride

You have been fooled by your fame and your pride, living there in the mountains of Petra, in the clefts of the rocks. But though you live among the peaks with the eagles, I will bring you down, says the Lord. Jeremiah 49:16 Life Recovery Bible

For years, a dear friend of mine has prayed for her family and church. Though she is known as a mighty prayer warrior, one problem attacked her recently that kept her in agony, day after day. Health problems riddled her body, causing anxiety to torment her mind. No victory came. While down at the altar one night, she asked me to pray for her. Later she confessed that as soon as I started praying at her request, peace came. What was keeping her from breaking through? Pride.

Satan uses deceit to cover our pride. Read the first phrase in the above verse again. "You have been fooled." We can spot pride in friends but, when it's in our lives, pride blinds us.

Pride follows success like low self-esteem comes after overeating.

When we aren't doing anything for God, Satan leaves us alone. If we stay lukewarm, we do the devil's job. When we climb the mountain top (teach, pray, witness), Satan again picks up his job and hits us with his best weapon—pride. Watch for symptoms when you eat healthy for several days. Be careful when someone compliments your weight loss. Watch out when you try to help others with the problem.

Regardless how high you fly, even as high as the eagles, the fall from pride can be devastating. When you falter, pray, but when you improve, pray even more.

Prayer: Lord, open my eyes so that I might see my true self and not the puffed-up version the devil shows me.

October 20

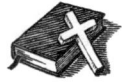

Time for My Check-Up

But let a man examine himself, and so let him eat of that bread, and drink of that cup. 1 Corinthians 11:28

Every year I go to three different doctors for my annual examinations. One doctor checks my eyes, one examines for recurring fibroid tumors and another checks my blood pressure and asthma. Even though I've had no recognizable problems in any of these areas, my doctors insist on seeing me. My family doctor will not refill my blood pressure medicine unless I come in. Why is that? Because they realize problems may present themselves to me unawares.

A frog who will not jump into a boiling pot of water because he senses danger will allow himself to swim in a pot while the fire underneath grows warmer to the point of boiling. An irritation or pain that gradually increases seems normal, so we can miss the signs.

That is also true spiritually. God suggested an examination of our actions and motives every time we take communion. We should periodically search for changes.

1. Have our attitudes darkened?
2. Do we do something we wouldn't have done in the past?
3. Are we craving food more often?
4. Is there a person or situation that causes anger?

Checking our outside—how much we weigh or how close we stay to our eating plan—isn't enough.

Is it time for a heart-issue check-up?

Prayer: Examine my heart today and put Your finger on anything that's not beneficial to my spiritual health.

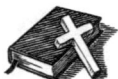

October 21

Be Assured

And the work of righteousness shall be peace and the effect of righteousness quietness and assurance forever. Isaiah 32:17

You may have heard the story of the little boy who asked Santa for a red wagon for Christmas. In excitement, he drove his new wagon too fast and a wheel came off.

He brought the wagon into his dad. "Please fix this."

"Lay it on my workshop," his dad said. "I'll fix it in a few minutes."

The boy put the wagon on the workshop counter, but then he decided that he could fix that wheel himself right now, so he took it to his room and tried screwing it on. It worked.

The next day, it came off again. The cycle repeated itself with the boy once again trying himself. He found a wire in his dad's tools and strung it between wheels. Off came the wheel again. Again, the boy brought it to his dad.

Days passed with similar results. Finally, the boy gave up. He plopped the wagon on the workbench and stomped to his room. That wagon was impossible to fix. He'd live without it.

That night, his dad came to his room and handed him the wagon. The wheels were tight and strong. Even the red finish shined with new brilliance. "Here, Son. I fixed it."

The boy's eyes widened. "Why didn't you fix it the first time I brought it to you?"

"Because," the dad said. "You never left it for me to fix."

Leave your sin, your filthy coat of unrighteousness, trouble and angst in God's hands. He promises quietness and peace in your soul.

Prayer: As I lay down my turmoil, give me the assurance of healing You promised.

October 22

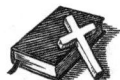

Yes, I Sin

If we confess our sins, he is faithful and just to forgive our sins, and to cleanse us from all unrighteousness. 1 John 1:9

I began to teach my weight recovery class with high hopes and low believability. Several years had passed since I had shed my weight, but something was wrong. Pounds crept back onto my body even while I stood and used myself as an example.

The class started small and decreased. My self-esteem hit bottom on a night when three other ladies joined me, each one suffering the "doldrums." I reviewed everything I'd taught, all firm, factual and uplifting. Why was the class unsuccessful?

The next week I prayed for guidance. God pointed out my sin of pride. Once again, God's number one culprit sunk another would-be teacher. I had started that class to try my written curriculum on others. My chest swelled at my accomplishment. I was eager to share it and then brag about it.

During the next session, my repentance genuine, I confessed my sin to the class. One dear friend rebuked me. She believed I was wallowing in low self-esteem. Again, the next week, I spent time in prayer and self-examination. God took me to the above verse. Though a low self-image had tormented me during much of my life, this wasn't that. This was sin, and I was right to confess it.

Good-meaning friends can tell you that you don't have sin to confess, but only you and God will know for sure. Verse 10 goes on to say if you think you don't sin, you deceive yourself. Don't ask a friend. Ask God. If he puts the finger on pride or anger or another sin, confess it. Only then can God continue to work in your life.

Prayer: Examine my life and let me know if You find any sin.

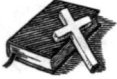

October 23

Follow Jesus

Jesus saith unto him, If I will that he tarry till I come, what is that to thee? Follow thou me. John:21:22.

At the time of this verse, Jesus is resurrected and appears to several of his disciples after they spent the night fishing without success. Jesus advised them to cast the net on the other side. They pulled in a load of fish by following Jesus' command.

Jesus then asked if they had eaten.

"No," they told him.

"Come and dine," Jesus said. He provided fish and bread for the hungry crew.

Peter suffered a guilty conscience since he had denied his Lord during the trial. He sought to seek Jesus' favor.

Yet, Jesus asked him three times if he loved Him.

Three times, Peter answered, "Yes."

Three times, Jesus told him to "follow me."

Like many of us, Peter compared what he might have to do with what God wanted of John. Jesus answered with the above verse.

When we begin a weight loss journey with Christ leading, we tend to compare our weight loss, our problems, our insights to others. Jesus requires we only follow Him. Even if the Lord allows your friend or your husband to lose twice as fast, what is that to you? Follow Jesus. When you stay the same for weeks, what does that have to do with it? Follow Jesus. If everything goes wrong to challenge your determination, who cares? Follow Jesus.

Prayer: Lead me today. I'll follow.

October 24

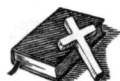

I Need Good Sense

For the Lord grants wisdom! His every word is a treasure of knowledge and understanding. He grants good sense to the godly—his saints. He is their shield, protecting them and guarding their pathway. Proverbs 2: 6,7 Life Recovery Bible

The meaning of insanity has been quoted as "doing the same thing over and over but expecting different results." In the realm of weight loss, that definition couldn't be more accurate.

Through the course of thirty years, I began one diet after another. Every time, I believed this one would bring the secret to success. I cut my calories to go on the diet and stuck to it completely for a period, but each time ended in failure. I would wait awhile and do the same thing again with perhaps a little different slant on the diet and, again, I'd expect success and receive despair.

When I put my weight problem in God's hands, two major differences stood out to me.

- I refused to diet, attempting solely to eat more fruits, vegetables and yogurt, stick with lean meats and whole grains, and limit almost to the point of cutting out any white sugar or flour.
- I followed the twelve steps of Overeaters Anonymous.

I gave up to God each day, knowing I could only make wise choices as long as He gave me the strength.

At my lowest, I did show definite signs of mental illness feeling the depths of depression to the point of planning suicide. God authors a sound mind. God gives us good sense, wisdom and knowledge. He guards our path.

Prayer: Give me good sense, today. I'm dependent on You.

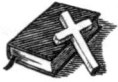

K.I.S.S. (Keep It Simple, Stupid)

Jesus replied, Foxes have holes and birds of the air have nests, but the Son of Man has no place to lay his head. Matthew 8:20 NIV

The religious leaders of the Jewish nation in Jesus' time were rich, famous and superior. They were set apart, looked up to, and answered the weighty questions of all things religious. Jesus came to the people as a simple man. On earth, he was poor, without even a home to call his own. He slept under the sky or sought refuge in humble abodes of friends.

When He spoke, His words held the authority of God, not merely the power of study, discussion, and debate. Jealousy wracked the leaders. They didn't understand His popularity. They preferred difficult rules to follow, where only they could interpret for the crowds. Jesus' message remained simple; understandable to a fisherman, a harlot, or a tax collector, without years of training.

I spent years looking for the perfect diet, the exact method of success, the plan that held the answer. The study provided me much wisdom in the field of nutrition and diet, but I kept an overweight body and besieged mind.

Like the religious leaders of Jesus' time, I tried to complicate the message. Like a tax accountant with the need to stay current on tax laws, I devoured each new thought the dieticians and doctors gave me to help me lose weight.

Jesus longs for us to "keep it simple." We know what to eat more of and what to leave off from our eating. The one thing we lack is lining up behind Jesus and letting Him lead.

Life and dieting can be difficult or simple. Which way are you doing it?

Prayer: Lead me according to Your simple plan today.

October 26

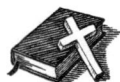

I'm Swamped

For wherever I am, though far away at the ends of the earth, I will cry to you for help. When my heart is faint and overwhelmed, lead me to the mighty, towering Rock of safety.
Psalms 61:2 Life Recovery Bible

There are times when I grow faint and overwhelmed.

- Finding myself plagued with more tasks than I can finish.
- Trying to be all things to all people.
- Fighting a desire to boost my energy when mine is depleted.

These are times when I give up and eat everything in sight.

Overeating slows our productivity and causes sluggishness and a bad attitude. Our salvation comes not from extra snacks or scrumptious desserts. In devouring these things, we put them in the place of God, but only the one true God can satisfy the weakness of our heart or restore the joy of our lives.

Rather than going to food—trying to fill ourselves by devouring more than our bodies can assimilate—turn to the Rock of our safety, and let God pour into that empty spot. When we give Him control, He leads us out of the rough time. As long as we hold onto the reins, stuffing in more and more food to ease the burden, we bog down deeper and deeper into misery and regret.

Prayer: When I go through an overwhelming time, lift my eyes to You.

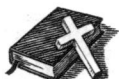

October 27

Remember the Alamo

But your eyes have seen all the great acts of the Lord which he did. Deuteronomy 11:7

I confess. I'm a Texas girl, born and bred on Texas history. In 1836, a small band of people gathered in the Alamo Mission, in what is now San Antonio, Texas. Their cause was all but defeated, as Mexican soldiers closed ranks around them. Nothing mattered to them except holding on to what they believed. Mexico defeated that group, killed everyone of them, but instead of stopping the revolution, it added fuel to Texan fortitude. From then on, when the men fought, they encouraged each other with the words: "Remember the Alamo." Men fought harder when they stopped to remember and allowed the emotion to motivate them.

In the verse above, Moses reminded the Israelites to remember what God had done for them, to recall the manna and the Red Sea crossing. Remembering motivated their trust.

When I falter now, I remember what "my eyes have seen" of God's power to control my eating. Often, the enemy closes in. I feel defeat on the horizon. But I've learned to look to the Lord.

Recall His mighty works on our behalf. The memories encourage us. He'll do it again if we call out and submit.

Prayer: May I never forget my Alamo or Red Sea weight loss experiences.

October 28

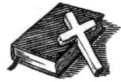

Hiding Place

Thou art my hiding place; thou shalt preserve me from trouble;
thou shalt compass me about with songs of deliverance.
Psalms 32:7

I love music. Until my asthma and medicines messed up my voice, I sang solos at church, for weddings and other events, and I sang in the church choir. I spent one semester in college aiming for a music major until I decided that was hard and switched to English. (Like that was easy. Ha!) I love the analogy of compassing me with songs of deliverance that David gave in this Psalm.

Temptation lured me into a wrong relationship with food. Food makes a faulty hiding place. Food exposes every weakness. How can it protect me when it only destroys?

My grandson loves to play the hide and seek game. He crouches behind a chair or stands behind a door. With peripheral vision, I spot him, but I pretend I don't so, when I pass, he can race to home base and beat me at the game. This is the way the devil wants me to hide. He fills me up with food, warps my view of life and adds other sins to my discredit. Because I hide in plain view but with clouded mind, he can hit me with defeat.

God's hiding place is secure. Trouble can not overcome me. When I read that verse, I treasure the idea of God shielding me with music. I envision angels circling me and singing, "My chains are gone."

Prayer: Lord, hide me today where I am safe.

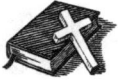

October 29

To Die or Not to Die

I tell you the truth, unless a kernel of wheat falls to the ground and dies, it remains only a single seed. But if it dies, it produces many seeds. John 12:24 NIV

To diet or not to diet,
That is not the question.
To unleash your inner giant
And kill selfish ambition

That's the dilemma we face
To restore focus and healing
It's through amazing grace
We're no longer ugly, greedy.

We must die to what we want
The spoiled, demanding child
Kill the inner man
God brings life undefiled.

It's not whether to diet
It's not eating certain foods
To commit to God's direction
Quit following our moods.

Janet K. Brown

Prayer: Today, I choose to die to self.

October 30

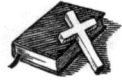

Forget Your Bad Times

Because thou shalt forget thy misery, and remember it as waters that pass away. Job. 11:16

I replay harsh words I've spoken or situations I've not handled with kindness. I turn on my internal DVD and watch it in the wee hours of the night. The words pop into my mind when I spot that individual. I feel inadequate then to say anything to anybody, afraid I'll wound others with my words.

Remembering the bad times:

- Cripples my ability to make friends
- Hampers me from openness and honesty
- Handicaps me as a wife, mother, child
- Impedes the advancement of my career
- Makes me see the worst in others
- Obstructs my Christian witness

BRINGS ME BACK TO OVEREATING.

I should remember:

- God healed my emotional disturbances.
- He forgave my past blunders.
- He healed my misery of self-defeating behavior.
- He asks that I remember it only as waters passed by.
- Dwelling on it hinders me from forgiving myself and soon I'll spiral back into the misery.

Prayer: Lord, help me never to dwell on the bad times, but only recall the good.

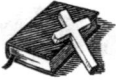

October 31

Is Jesus Your Plumb Line?

As you have therefore received Christ Jesus, the Lord, walk (regulate your lives and conduct yourselves) in union with and conformity to Him. Colossians 2:6 TAB

My husband won't let me anywhere near a paint brush. I end up with the floor, furniture, and myself covered with paint, along with an occasional dusting on the wall. So, a few years ago, when we picked out new wallpaper, it was understood that he would be the one to hang it, not me. I watch.

"I love hard work. I can watch it all day." Anonymous.

Before my husband added the glue to the backside of the paper, he hung what looked like a long string at the corner of the two walls from the ceiling. At the bottom of the string was a metal weight. Where the metal fell hung almost an inch away from the adjacent wall. "They didn't use a plumb line when attaching these two walls," he said.

Most of you know enough about building to know the reason for using a plumb bob. This keeps the builder working in a straight line. Our eyes mislead us. What looks the exact distance is proven wrong. By doing this, my husband made adjustments and the wallpaper came out even.

I got to thinking about how we go along matching our conduct and decisions with what the Bible teaches. We make choices according to what seems right but, after awhile, if we don't continually study the "plumb line" (God's Word), we get off line.

So it is with our lives. I eat sweets one day—not a bad thing—but I crave them for a week, and sometimes I succumb again and again. I can take one tiny turn, when I don't ask God's guidance, and it throws me off more and more.

Prayer: Lord, remind me to use You for my life's plumb line.

November 1

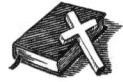

God's Mercy

*And if anyone's name was not found recorded in the Book of Life,
he was thrown into the Lake of Fire.*
Revelations 20:15 Life Recovery Bible

God offers unmerited favor on his creation (people). Salvation comes when we accept His gift.

We also receive deliverance from food addiction by reaching out and laying hold of His mercy. We don't deserve it. We did nothing to warrant it. We did, in fact, rebel against His commands. We betrayed His sacrifice. We fell short of His desire for us. Inventory of our sin finds us wanting. We hate what we have become.

I disliked the examination. It revealed anger, resentment, envy, self pity, and disobedience. My mind told me I needed to make myself good enough for God, but that wasn't possible.

Here's my experience. I needed to lose weight. I needed to take the emphasis off the desirable foods that set my heart to pounding, my mouth to watering. My internal conversations went like this. "After **I** set my will power. After **I** whip my body into control. After **I** make myself lose weight. Then, I'll repent." Are these words familiar?

This too was sin. This was pride. This was refusing God's mercy.

As humiliating as it is, it is best to take our inventory now. When we face our ineptitude, when we can accept His mercy with gratitude because, now, it's all God. As Revelation tells us, God's inventory is coming, but He only looks to see if there is anything in our lives uncovered by Jesus' blood.

Prayer: Thankfulness to God eliminates my sin.

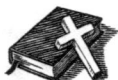

November 2

Tune In

But they hearkened not, nor inclined their ear, but walked in the counsels and in the imagination of their evil heart, and went backward and not forward. Jeremiah 7:24

I meet with a group of three women friends. Our belief in Christ and our desire to exercise for health brought us together years ago. On our lunch breaks, we walked around the inside edge of our mall for exercise. One by one, each woman retired and quit walking. Anxious to keep our friendship strong, I called them and arranged to meet for lunch.

All four of us keep up with Facebook. A month after our first luncheon, one of the group called. "I've sent you many messages on Facebook, but you haven't responded. We're meeting at lunch today. Can you come?"

With prior notice, I could've planned better, but at the last minute, I couldn't go. I missed a blessing. My friend reached out to me with messages several times, but I failed to hear.

Every day a radio station plays uplifting music but we don't receive it if we don't tune the set to the frequency. God speaks to us. He directs His wisdom to a listening audience. He broadcasts a signal to each believer. But unless we "incline our ear" or tune in to His messages, we will not hear. We will not respond. We will miss the blessing of His strength and direction.

Prayer: Talk to me, Lord. I'll strive to tune in to Your Words.

November 3

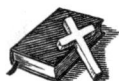

Pride Brings Craziness

The king spake, and said, Is not this great Babylon, that I have built for the house of the kingdom by the might of my power, and for the honour of my majesty? While the word was in the king's mouth, there fell a voice from heaven, saying, "O king Nebuchadnezzar, to thee it is spoken; The kingdom is departed from thee." Daniel 4:30,31

God gave us an example of pride ending in defeat. The verse above shows the Babylonian king, puffed up with pride for all his accomplishment, and then God's view of the situation.

God allowed and provided Nebuchadnezzar's wealth and might. When he took all glory for himself, God moved in and showed how weak the king really was. Nebuchadnezzar fell into insanity, not remembering even his name. He lived in his madness in fields with the animals until God brought him back to awareness and returned him to his kingdom.

This time, Nebuchadnezzar called out, "His dominion is an everlasting dominion. And His kingdom is from generation to generation." (Daniel 4:34)

Oftentimes, we too must learn that pride brings craziness. Our kingdom may be our family, our career, our possessions, even our work at church. We believe we're indispensable, our title is something to be coveted. We will our families to act perfectly. We direct the play of our lives.

God sees the reality. He awaits our breakdown. For some of us, it shows up in a food binge, or a flash of anger, or a total collapse, or all three. When the pride is gone, God picks up the pieces and restores our mental, physical, and spiritual health. Some of us fall faster than others, but when we do, God is there.

Prayer: Forgive my pride. Heal my craziness. Restore my kingdom.

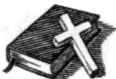

November 4

A Private Affair

Behold thou desirest truth in the inward parts; and in the hidden part thou shall make me to know wisdom. Psalms 51:6

Some things about us we show to no one, not even our husbands, best friends, or other relatives. Our compulsion to overeat is a private affair. We might eat too much at a party or get-together, but those times, when we get lost in a bag of candy or a dozen donuts, we act in hiding, alone.

"The most difficult part in being honest is confessing. Ego becomes a stumbling block, as does fear of hurting our image." *Partners in Prayer* by John Maxwell.

God wants truth even in our private times.

When we binge, we must confess. Some Christian congragations believe in a private confessional with the pastor. Twelve-step programs demand confession to a sponsor or a trusted friend. Standing before the church or a class to confess isn't required, but honesty before at least one other person pulls that ugly secret out of hiding where God's light can shine on it. Secrets evaporate in the sunshine of God's love.

Neither should it be a private affair when God heals. Bring that into the open. We must testify, to everyone who might benefit, that Jesus healed our emotions and replaced our compulsion for food with Him.

Prayer: Today, Help me live in openness before God and another person.

November 5

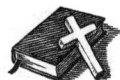

Is Your Love Selfish?

Charity suffereth long, and is kind; charity envieth not; charity vaunteth not itself; is not puffed up. 1 Corinthians 13:4

When our systems clear from overeating sugar and fried foods, sanity returns. God can't speak well to a mind bogged down in food overload. God speaks to a newly-cleared mind of other pesky problems plaguing our work, hampering our witness.

Has God put His finger on the quality of your love?

A compulsive overeater can be selfish. It's all about us. How does our family reflect on us? What can our friends do for us? If our children fall short of our expectations, what does that make us look like? Do we attempt to control friends and families, maybe even our church or jobs, to make us look more pious? Do you manipulate your husband or children to get your own way? Do you begrudge coworkers or other church workers the praise they receive? Is there an element of selfishness in your love?

The Life Recovery Bible states the above verse and verse five as: "Love is very patient and kind, never jealous or envious, never boastful or proud, never haughty or selfish or rude. Love does not demand its own way. It is not irritable or touchy. It does not hold grudges and will hardly even notice when others do it wrong."

God asks us to measure our love against His way of loving. Many of us fall short.

Prayer: Lord, teach me to love like You do.

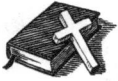

November 6

Time to Renew

But they that wait upon the Lord shall renew their strength; they shall mount up with wings as eagles, they shall run, and not be weary; and they shall walk, and not faint. Isaiah 40:31

We're newer people than we were ten years ago. Physically, each cell in our body renews every seven to ten years. This is God's plan to restore, replenish, and revitalize, so that we can live for decades. God built our bodies as living miracles.

For years, it's been thought that brain cells don't regenerate. Now, new studies indicate they do. Why not? God thought of everything else.

Spiritual renewal must also take place for God's children who wish to continue the Christian walk for life. In God's Word, He explains how we renew strength: Wait for God.

None of us like to wait. We want what we want, and we want it now. This is no more true than in losing weight. Though we spent years overweight, we desire a svelte body in two weeks. Though we've eaten everything in sight for weeks, we want to re-lose the weight in two days.

God's way of losing weight is slow, but it is permanent and restores health. He begins with emotional healing, moves on to lifestyle changes, and finishes with your total submission to Him. That takes time.

When impatience overtakes us, we should remember the familiar verse above. If we wait on God, we gain strength to fly, walk and not faint.

Prayer: Help me wait for You, Lord.

November 7

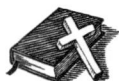

God's Caffeine

To whom he said, This is the rest wherewith ye may cause the weary to rest; and this is the refreshing; yet they would not hear. Isaiah 28:12

Stress overcomes us when we continually live in a fight-or-flight mode with no rest or downtime to replenish ourselves, to refuel our bodies and strengthen our minds. When we have too little sleep or see too much work to do, many of us use food as if it were caffeine. Some does contain caffeine but, more often than not, it's just a break we need—so we eat. Too much food can overload our senses causing DUI-type car wrecks, weight gain, inability to concentrate on our jobs, and/or thoughtless actions.

We need *God's* caffeine:

C onfidence

A wesome power

F avor

F ight

E nergy

I nner peace

N ap

E ffectiveness

Only God can give enough rest or energy to accomplish our tasks without the side effects. Food in excess can be as danger-ous to our plans as alcohol or as deadly as poison, or as sleep-depriving as energy drinks.

Prayer: Energize me with the rest of Jesus.

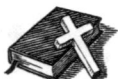

November 8

Begin Now On This Day

. . . behold, now is the accepted time; behold, now is the day of salvation. 2 Corinthians 6:2b

A lifetime of dieting teaches us that Monday is the day to begin. Procrastination hinders all opportunity for growth. Paul directs us in the verse above that *today* is the day to turn your life to Christ.

Today is the day to give your food addiction to Christ. Start now, whether it's noon or nine in the evening.

The devil works around the clock to block our path to God. If he can delay our freedom, he's won another round in the battle. Even if we're working for God, praying and doing our best to serve Him, overeating weakens our witness and wilts our effectiveness.

Many may not agree, but think about it. Is this a situation you need to pray about and work out with the Lord? What if the addiction were drugs? Would it then be suitable to wait until Monday to gain your freedom?

I spent years starting on Monday, stopping by Wednesday and starting on another Monday. Does this resonate with you?

What if we start after the piece of cheesecake and ask God to take over our weakness now? I never received God's healing until I was willing to stop and make a one-eighty right then, even if I was on vacation.

Prayer: Lord, let NOW be my time for freedom. Take over,
now.

November 9

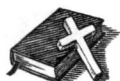

Feasts and Fasts

You new moons and your appointed feasts my soul hateth; they are a trouble unto me; I am weary to bear them. Isaiah 1:14

I purchase new foods, study the new plan, and prepare the way for an elaborate dive into a new me. This will be the one, the diet to end all diets. I'm hyped up to go all the way. I'm like a cheerleader for a football team.

Go, fight, lose!

The night before we begin the "change" in our lives, we stop to buy a luscious treat, we go to a restaurant for dinner and choose a fattening entree, then we follow-up with a pint of ice cream before midnight of the DAY.

Do we stop to wonder what God thinks about all our plans? He told the Israelites He hated their festivals and feasts. Why? Because they left Him out. It was all a sham, an outward ritual that meant nothing.

If you had just forty-eight hours left to live, how would you spend them?

Will Rogers said: *"One at a time!"*

Don't start a new diet. Start a new dedication, and do it one day at a time.

Prayer: I refuse to start today on my own. Guide me, Lord.

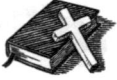

November 10

Where Is Your Confidence?

In the fear of the Lord is strong confidence; and his children shall have a place of refuge. The fear of the Lord is a fountain of life, to depart from the snares of death. Proverbs 14: 26,27

Look at the Life Recovery Bible for this verse:
Reverence for God gives a man deep strength, his children have a place of refuge and security. Reverence for the Lord is a fountain of life; its waters keep a man from death.

Too much food hampers your health. An eating disease can ultimately bring death. Eating healthy, God-given foods provides a good physical life, a fountain of youth. Our children and grandchildren reap the blessings of our help and wisdom for years. What is it that brings about this miracle? Fear (reverence) for God.

Where's your confidence?

Hollywood, doctors, new diet, a gym?

God?

We say, "It's impossible."

God says, "All things are possible through me."

We say, "I can't go on."

God says, "My grace is sufficient."

Prayer: I lay prostrate before my God. Without You, I'm doomed.

November 11

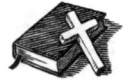

Willingness

For if there be first a willing mind, it is accepted according to that a man hath, and not according to that he hath not.
2 Corinthians 8:12

This verse talks about a willing mind toward giving. God provides the example of the tithe, so everyone gives equally, "according to what a man hath." God requires a willing mind to follow Him in total obedience, whether in charity or in defeating addiction.

He may bring on more than we can handle by ourselves, but He never allows more temptation than we, with his help, can handle. His escape route involves our submission, not our white-knuckle will power. If we were strong enough within ourselves to conquer food compulsion, we wouldn't need God—but we can't.

"Insane people are always sure that they are fine. It is only the sane people who are willing to admit that they are crazy." Nora Ephron, screenwriter and director

Compulsive overeaters are crazy. Do you have a willing mind to commit your actions, thoughts and hopes to God? He requires nothing less, and nothing more.

Prayer: Make me more willing.

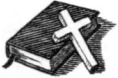

November 12

Deliver Me From Disdain and Condescension

The Pharisee stood and prayed thus with himself, God, I thank thee, that I am not as other men are, extortionists, unjust, adulterers, or even as this publican. Luke 18:11

Once, I rode an elevator with two overweight friends. They admired my weight loss. I preened and grinned like a peacock on parade. "It's hard work, but you just have to do it." Immediately, conviction heated my cheeks, and I fumbled for words of apology. In years past, my body was more bloated with fat than theirs, yet my words condemned them and hurt their feelings.

We look at a person heavier than ourselves and think how grateful we are not to be that big. When another Christian makes a scene about something they disagree with, we congratulate ourselves for keeping our tempers.

God uses His Word as the ruler to measure our actions one at a time. He checks His commands versus our obedience. He judges the skinny person against themselves. Could there be factors such as illness that keeps them thin? Do we wallow in pride while the skinny person obeys Christ?

Jesus tells us the Pharisee in the above verse went away unjustified, while the lowly publican who prayed, "Lord, forgive me, a sinner," went away cleansed.

God looks on the individual heart. After God heals us and helps us lose weight, we must continue to seek His mind and compassion, *less we lose what we have gained, and gain what we have lost.*

Prayer: Deliver me from a disdainful, hurtful attitude.

November 13

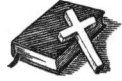

Spoiled Brat

If any man will do his will, he shall know of the doctrine, whether it be of God, or whether I speak of myself. John 7:17

Last spring break, my husband and I took our grandsons out to eat. The younger boy ordered an enchilada with chili sauce. When the food was delivered, the sauce was green. Our grandson turned up his nose. He not only refused to eat it, he pouted and kicked his legs. The server obliged with a red chili sauce, then a cheese sauce. Nothing pleased the young boy.

"No, I don't want it," he squealed.

His actions ruined the entire evening for us and his brother. In his defense, he apologized later and we've since taken him out for a pleasurable dinner.

We have all witnessed our children or those of other people playing the part of spoiled brat. None of us like the mentality.

Does God view us as spoiled brats at times?

What is a "spoiled brat?"

Is it not someone who demands his or her own way? Who pouts and screams when he doesn't get his way? Is it not a selfish response?

"Dwight L Moody spoke to us simply and briefly using John 7:17 . . . . There in the quiet, without anyone knowing what was going on, I gave myself to God, my whole mind, heart and body; and I meant it." Henry Wright

If we want to know God's will, God will open our minds to know. We must be willing to accept it, even if it's "green," even if God's will conflicts with what we want. Follow it. Refuse to act like a spoiled brat. Submit to a better way.

Prayer: Open my eyes, soften my heart, direct my steps.

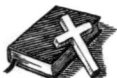

November 14

Bewitched and Bewildered

O foolish Galatians, who hath bewitched you that ye should not obey the truth, before whose eyes Jesus Christ hath been evidently set forth, crucified among you? Galatians 3:1

When my mother was young, she loved a song called "Bewitched and Bewildered." When my children were young, we enjoyed together reruns of a TV series called "Bewitched." The term intrigues us. *Webster's New World Dictionary* defines bewitch as "to cast a spell over or to attract or delight greatly." Their definition of bewildered is "to puzzle or confuse hopelessly."

In the verse above, Paul writes a letter to the church of Galatia asking who confused or cast a spell on them. When we give our hearts to Jesus Christ crucified, it is evident to us the Word is truth and, therefore, we obey.

He is our Savior, but is He king over our lives?

"The Lord's Prayer is not as some fancy—the easiest, the most natural of all devout utterances. It may be committed to MEMORY quickly, but it is slowly learned by HEART." Anonymous

"Thy kingdom come, thy will be done."

Does food bewitch us? Does resentment turn us from what's evident? Is it time to face the truth?

Prayer: Protect my mind from bewitchment.

November 15

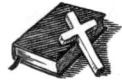

Elijah, Jonah, and Me

But he himself went a day's journey into the wilderness, and came and sat down under a juniper tree; and he requested for himself that he might die; and said, It is enough, now, O Lord, take away my life for I am not better than my fathers.
1 Kings 19:4

Elijah, wrestled with depression. After a major victory for God when he stood against all the prophets of Ba`al, King Ahab threatened Elijah's life. This mighty prophet of God slipped into depression to the point of wanting to die, to give up because he feared what laid ahead of him. He didn't know if he could keep doing what he needed to do.

Therefore, now, O Lord, take, I beseech thee, my life from me; for it is better for me to die than to live. Jonah 4:3

Jonah preached to the Ninevites, and they repented before God. This prophet was so reluctant to preach the Word to his enemies, he ran from God. God prepared a big fish to bring Jonah back to the mission. Faithful to His Word, God spared the enemy city because they turned to Him. Jonah got mad at God and begged to die.

"I sat out to see how much I could stuff in my mouth that tasted good. On Sunday morning, I cried and cried. I had no answer, no avenue of coping. I decided Sunday evening to eat, but I had little in my house to overdose on. I tried pear preserves and bread, bananas, graham crackers, peanuts. Nothing helped."

That quote comes from an old journal of mine. Depression affects Godly men and us. God is the only satisfaction to be found in life, the only cure to depression.

Prayer: Help me look to You for my coping ability.

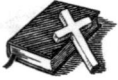

November 16

This Tastes Good.

You provide delicious food for me in the presence of my enemies.
You have welcomed me as your guest; blessings overflow.
Psalms 23: 5 Life Recovery Bible

God spreads a table for us in the midst of others who overeat. God offers good tasting foods to satisfy our desires.

During Thanksgiving and Christmas holidays, the majority of people give themselves permission to indulge in more food and richer delights than any other time of year. This can be a nightmare for an individual who can't control food. We're tempted to give in to obsessive desires. We sit at the table with others who load their plates (our enemies, if you will), but even here, God provides delicious food (turkey, fruit salad, steamed veggies) and great blessings.

Remember at these times to choose wisely. Use the modified motto: "What would Jesus eat?" He provided vegetables, fruits, grains and meats to bless our appetites. He gives us strength to control man's overindulgence in refined sugars and rich buttery additions. We can eat and feel blessed.

Prayer: Thank you, Lord, for Your delicious food that truly
satisfies without bloating.

November 17

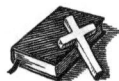

Beginning Anew

He openeth also their ear to discipline, and commandeth that they return from iniquity. Job 36:10

Beginning anew is hard. There's something about doing a job over again that increases its difficulty. Computers mess up and lose data. Many of us have been forced to enter facts and figures for the second time because of a hard-drive crash. What seamstress has not finished a dress only to find she put the top on backwards, needed to rip it out, and start from scratch? Executives offer a plan for next year's expansion, only to find a flaw and need to begin again.

"Don't let life discourage you; everyone who got where he is had to begin where he was." Richard L. Evans

Don't be defeated when you regain weight that you agonized over losing. The facts don't change. You start from where you are. The walk with God constantly changes. This weight loss will not duplicate the last one. We must return from the evil place. We must open our ears to God's discipline. If God commands it, He will journey with us.

Prayer: Here I am again, Lord. Lead me on a fresh path.

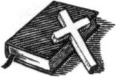

November 18

Uncultivated Ground

Sow for yourselves according to righteousness (uprightness and right standing with God); reap according to mercy and loving-kindness. Break up your uncultivated ground, for it is time to seek the Lord, to inquire for and of Him, and to require His favor, till He comes and teaches you righteousness and rains His righteous gift of salvation upon you. Hosea 10:12 TAB

All good things in life require persistence. A salesman who gives up after the first "No" he receives will never succeed. When a farmer's crop wilts in the field, he plows it back into the ground and prepares the soil, working extra hard to get ready for the next season. My husband is a realtor. One year, it seemed every contract he wrote fell through before one made it to sale. "It happens," he says.

When I started submitting the stories I wrote to publishers, I faced five years of rejection. Each rejection letter hurt. At first, I considered quitting, but I took another course, I went to a writer's conference, I cultivated new ground, and submitted a new story.

The life of a compulsive overeater compels us to sow new seeds, to break up uncultivated ground, to try new methods. Learning to lean on God for a simple thing like the food we eat takes time and work. Now is not the time to stop. Now is the time to **sow, reap, break up, seek, inquire** until He sends the rains of rewarding repairs.

"This is the highest wisdom that I own, freedom and life are earned by those alone who conquer them each day anew." Johann Wolfgang Von Goethe, German playwright, poet, and novelist

Prayer: I seek of You, Lord, the ability to begin again.

November 19

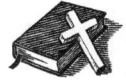

Persistence

Pray all the time. Ask God for anything in line with the Holy Spirit's wishes. Plead with him, reminding him of your needs, and keep praying earnestly for all Christians everywhere.
Ephesians 6:18

My son-in-law is a high school baseball and football coach. He's good at inspiring young men to excellence and, because of that, many times his team wins. He's taken several teams to the state baseball finals near Austin, Texas. During the baseball season, his players tell of the motivational calls they receive every morning.

Some teams falter. Not all win even most of the time. Some lose a lot. The day after a heart-breaking loss, my son-in-law stands before these defeated young men. He claps his hands. His voice reverberates with excitement. "Shake it off, men. We've got great things ahead. The next game, we will be unshakeable."

I stand in awe of his ability to "shake it off" and stay positive, but that's his job. He must, or he'd never win again. A few minutes after a rough loss, reporters hit him with, "What did you do wrong?" His favorite expression is: "We're okay."

As compulsive overeaters, or food addicts, we fall on our faces with stupid errors, and heart-rending mistakes. Don't be afraid to remind God of your needs. He tells us to plead with Him, to not quit praying every day.

Look in the mirror right now and say, "You're okay" because you are.

Prayer: Lord, it's me again. I need help. I can't do it. With You, I'm okay.

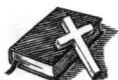

November 20

Journal On Your Journey

And the Lord answered me and said, Write the vision and engrave it so plainly upon tablets that everyone who passes may [be able to]read [it easily and quickly] as he hastens by.
Habakkuk 2:2 TAB

I love writing. Since my junior high school days, I have written something every day, so keeping a journal of my journey wasn't difficult.

For some, writing is a chore, they shy away from it like yellow fever. God created us as body, mind, and spirit. Our three parts intertwine and reinforce each other. Something about commissioning our hands to write ignites our minds to think and our spirits to rise. Writing can take different forms.

- Tracking everything we eat in a day.
- Writing elaborate journals of what we think, what we do, or difficulties we face.
- Tweeting a motivational thought each day.
- Posting on Facebook something we learned about life, or eating, or ourselves.
- Putting pen to paper when we're angry and writing a letter condemning the one who made us mad. (But throw it away, don't give it to them.)
- Recording something we found made us eat what we shouldn't.
- Reading what we wrote a week ago, or a month ago, and responding to it with new vision.
- Keep a praise journal for answered prayers.

Think of other ways to write. Pick what works. We're all different people, so it many methods may minister from one person to another. Writing the vision as God asked Habakkuk to do can enforce our healing, and remove our addiction.

Prayer: Lead me to journal as You lead me on my journey to health.

November 21

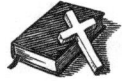

God's Portion Control

Then said the Lord unto Moses, Behold, I will rain bread from heaven for you, and the people shall go out and gather a certain rate every day, that I may prove them, whether they will walk in my law, or no. Exodus 16:4

God provides food
And that is abundant.
He gives us free will
Obedience, redundant.

Does He watch and decide
If we follow direction?
The portion He gives
Allows for defection.

Obedience—not forced
He wants love given freely.
We hold the fork
But, feel His love keenly

What is our choice? God watches as He did with the Israelites to see whether we will follow His rules without murmuring or complaining. He never makes us. He wants us to choose His will, His love, His way with freedom.

Prayer: Today, I choose God over food.

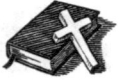

My World is Moving Fast and Veering out of My Grasp

Cast thy burden upon the Lord, and he shall sustain thee, he shall never suffer the righteous to be moved. Psalms 55:22

Certain times in our lives rush us into almost oblivion. Thinking about what we should eat is the last thing on our minds. Remember weeks of grief after losing a loved one because of death. Think about those times of good-byes to a child moving away or even going to war. Other happier times infect our need to eat healthy; family reunions, preparing and enjoying the wedding of a child, moving to a new home. When a compulsive overeater thinks of times like this in life, we give into our addiction thinking we have no choice.

God tells us to cast our burdens on Him. He will sustain us. (He will provide healthy fare from which to choose and detour your need so that you relish the veggies and fruits or He can bring about a hunger for lean proteins. Our job is to allow God to move in all circumstances, to walk with us down every path.

I'm reminded of a story I read about a little girl:

One day, a little girl whispered to her Sunday school teacher, "Sometimes Jesus comes and walks with me."

"Where, dear?" the teacher asked.

"Oh, just anywhere I am—on the sidewalk, in school, in our yard."

"And what do you do when Jesus walks with you?"

Instantly came the reply, "I just move over and make room for Him to walk close to me."

Are you making room for Jesus even when your life is moving fast, wherever you are?

Prayer: I want You to walk with me today. I pray I'll make room.

November 23

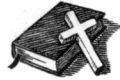

Thy Will, Not Mine

Thy kingdom come, Thy will be done in earth, as it is in heaven.
Matthew 6:10

How many times do we say these lines from the Lord's prayer and think about what they mean? In heaven, angels obey without question, without thinking, without rebellion. When we pray the words above, we ask that humans (us) follow that same system.

God gave us a free will, a mind of our own. He could've formed us like robots, and then we would follow His desires. God wanted us to love Him *of our own free will.* As a parent, I love when my children think of something to give me or do for me that I didn't ask, maybe never even thought of, and they do it because they love me. God is like that.

Obeying His commands tells God we love Him.

Discard rebellion.

Eliminate anger

Do away with hate.

His will be done.

"He has a right to interrupt your life. He is Lord. When you accepted Him as Lord, you gave Him the right to help Himself to your life anytime He wants." Henry Blackaby

The military teaches soldiers to jump when a command is given.

Prayer: Lord, make me a good soldier. Thy will, not mine.

327

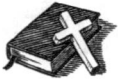

November 24

Refocus

And Peter answered him and said Lord, if it be thou, bid me come unto thee on the water. And he said, 'Come.' And when Peter was come down out of the ship, he walked on the water, to go to Jesus. But when he saw the wind boisterous, he was afraid, and beginning to sink, he cried, saying, Lord, save me. And immediately Jesus stretched forth his hand and caught him, and said unto him, 'O thou of little faith, wherefore didst thou doubt?'
Matthew 14:28-31

Jesus worked a miracle here according to this familiar story. Pete, also lived a miracle for a moment until he doubted. Though this story teaches us that we, like Peter, can work miracles in Jesus' power, the main lesson in the story is Peter's failure. Why did he fail? And what did he do then?

God works miracles of healing in our lives. He has in the past and will continue to do so. Food loses its luster when we focus on Christ. The more we study His word, pray and meditate on Jesus, the more our hunger for Him intensifies. When we spend less time with God, our hunger for food grows.

God replaces food. Or food supersedes God. Our choice.

If we find ourselves constantly battling a desire to overeat and can no longer leave half our meal on the plate, we must REFOCUS.

We must do it now. Not tomorrow morning. Not next Monday. Now. We must get to our knees, and ask God to help us look in the right place. Peter failed when he looked at the water. Peter succeeded when he looked back to Jesus. So can we.

Prayer: Fill my mind and heart today so there's no room for a substitute.

November 25

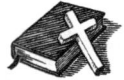

Moderation

Let your moderation be known unto all men. The Lord is at hand.
Philippians 4:5

When I read the above, it dawns on me that I have never connected the two sentences in that verse. We quote, "Let your moderation be known unto all men." We roll our eyes and think how hard that command is for us to keep. America is a country of excess or lack.

We work too much, we play video games too often, and we super-size our eating.

We sleep too little, spend too little time with our families, and don't say "thank you" nearly enough.

Moderation is a foreign word to most modern-day Americans.

The forgotten second sentence reminds us that though God desires from us moderation, He stands ready to add strength to our weakness, restraint to our imbalance, and abundance to our deficiency.

Our emotional turmoil sends us up and down like a runaway horse or a off-the-track roller coaster. Excessive emotion causes us to eat as if food could add balm to our wounds. When we're caught in that tug-of-war between anger and guilt, *God is at hand.*

Prayer: Soothe my hurts, assuage my guilt, take over my mind.

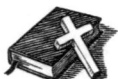

November 26

Learning Recovery

I know how to live on almost nothing or with everything. I have learned the secret of contentment in every situation, whether it be a full stomach or hunger, plenty or want; for I can do everything God asks me to do with the help of Christ.
Philippians 4:12,13 Life Recovery Bible

The National Health and Nutrition Survey in 2004 told us 133.6 million (66%) adult Americans were obese or overweight. A Purdue University study indicates conservative churches such as Southern Baptists, Assembly of God and Church of God fight this battle more often. Richard Kreider of Baylor University gives further insight into this. These denominations "avoid dancing, tobacco and alcohol, but give no guidelines for overeating." He goes on to say our churches more often attract with food, not action events.

Overeaters cope with church potlucks and dessert parties. We abstain from alcohol but laugh about big stomachs. We read about gluttony in the Bible without drawing a parallel to us. We overeat or we give up church functions altogether.

Last night, at a church party, my friend ate before she came, then sat with us while we ate. If you find yourself doing this, remember it can deprive you of being part of the group, even when there, and make you lonely, detached, and forlorn.

We must fit into all situations. Recovery demands a learning process. Losing a few pounds doesn't make us an expert.

The process of recovery is a time of learning to find serenity while also accepting life as it is. Life isn't fair; it isn't predictable, or controllable; it can be wonderfully rich in some ways and terribly difficult in others. Life Recovery Bible pg. 1329

Prayer: Teach me recovery as I pass through life's ups and downs.

November 27

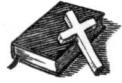

Where's My Focus?

Then Mary took about a pint of pure nard, an expensive perfume; she poured it on Jesus' feet and wiped his feet with her hair.
John 12:2 NIV

Compulsive overeaters turn inward. At one time my motto—though I wouldn't admit it—was "It's all about me." Feeling sorry for myself exacerbated my eating, and eating increased my low self-esteem. The vicious cycle churned in my mind and spiraled to lower depths with each day. At one point in my life, even though I had a faithful husband and three precious daughters, I could see nothing worthwhile to my life. Feeling empty and void of any good thing, I truly believed my family would be better off without me.

I wrote this devotion at Christmas time. I just returned from stuffing stockings for under-privileged children. My mouth sings and my heart feels weightless. My mind focuses on others, not myself. I feel good about helping someone.

In chapter twelve of John, Mary loved Jesus and she longed to show Him how much she cared. The only thing she could think of was to break open her perfume, which was possibly the only thing of value she owned, and anoint Jesus' feet. Many thought that action foolish. Once a friend thought I was crazy for picking up a mentally-challenged lady and bringing her to Bible study. This sweet lady didn't seem to know what we were saying and added nothing to the conversation. But, in doing this, my mind stayed on her, not me.

Do what you can. Do what God leads you to do. Focus on someone besides yourself. God will worry about your food.

Prayer: Lord, show me what You'd have me do today to encourage or help another soul.

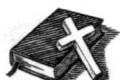

November 28

Drink the Water

You are a fountain [springing up] in a garden, a well of living waters, and flowing streams from Lebanon.
Song of Solomon 4:15

Our bodies are 70-75% water. The human brain is about 85%, and our bones are between 10 to 15% water. Water provides the best diet aid known to man. Its many advantages are:
- Suppresses the appetite.
- Reduces sodium buildup.
- Helps maintain muscle tone.
- Eliminates waste and toxins.
- Relieves fluid retention.
- Reduces fat deposits.
- Keeps kidneys and liver functioning properly.
- Alleviates common ailments such as allergies, asthma, depression, high blood pressure, diabetes, headaches, chronic fatigue syndrome, colitis, alcohol dependency, lower back pain, neck pain, and urinary tract infections.
- Decreases wrinkles, dry and itchy skin, and nosebleeds.

The average adult loses 2.5 liters of water daily, so it must constantly be replenished.

Jesus is our Savior, our King, and the Lover of our Souls. Solomon likens Him unto a fountain of water springing up and streaming through the gardens of our minds. Our spiritual lives wither and die without repeated replenishment from the fountain that only Jesus supplies. Our ability to do God's work, to refrain from overeating, to renew our commitment, to obey God comes through daily soaking in the stream of *living water*.

God created us to require both physical and spiritual water.

Prayer: Lord, cleanse me and saturate me with Your fountain of life.

November 29

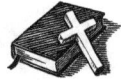

Service Required

Who comforts (consoles and encourages) us in every trouble (calamity and affliction), so that we may also be able to comfort (console and encourage) those who are in any kind of trouble or distress, with the comfort (consolation and encouragement) with which we ourselves are comforted (consoled and encouraged) by God. 2 Corinthians 1:4 TAB

One of the twelve steps most often forgotten or neglected is number 12, which says "Having had a spiritual awakening as the result of these steps, we tried to carry this message to alcoholics, and to practice these principles in all our affairs." Alcoholics Anonymous.

Our recovery from overeating or any compulsion comes through following all the steps. God requires for us to pass on what we have received. He encourages us; we are to encourage others.

Service to others while still bogged down in overeating and emotional turbulence is required. Daily, we must ask ourselves:

Who have we encouraged today?

Who have we prayed for today?

What have we done to help a fellow addict?

"God does not comfort us to make us comfortable but to make us comforters." Gregory L. Jantz, Ph.D

Prayer: Keep me sensitive to those still tormented with an overeating compulsion.

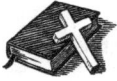

November 30

Sing

Make a joyful noise unto the Lord, all ye lands. Serve the Lord with gladness; come before his presence with singing.
Psalms 100:1,2

During the season of Thanksgiving, more than any time of the year, we take time to step back and praise God for all He's done. One of the blessings of the season at our church is the special music.

When I was younger, I sang solos and participated in church choirs. Illness and medications ruined my voice for a couple of years and caused my singing to cease. I still love singing, but I let others stand in front to lead.

Music delights the soul and draws us into a closer relationship with God. A less-than-great voice should never keep us from singing praise to Him. Music heightens our praises, our prayers, our altar time, and our worship.

Music can also restore equilibrium to a troubled mind. Some days we start the day struggling. Every chore becomes a battle. Turmoil can dim, emotions can still, craving can lessen when we sing or listen to singing.

There's a reason David, through the inspiration of God, advises us to "come into His presence with singing."

Prayer: Remind me of a song of love to sing today.

December 1

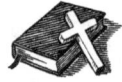

Mistakes or Miracles

Know ye that the Lord, he is God, it is he that hath made us, and not we ourselves; we are his people and the sheep of his pasture.
Psalms 100:3

A few years ago, a favorite saying was: "God don't make no junk." We must remember how we came to be. The quiet geek, the boisterous jock, the back-stabbing corporate-climber; God made them all. I have a friend known for her quirky personality. She offends some by her blunt remarks, yet her heart seeks God, her motives stay pure. She studies His Word with an aggression that outranks many preachers.

My friend points out, "God gave me this strange sense of humor along with my oft-intimidating personality. I figure He intends me to use it for Him."

She does so by opening her house for Bible studies, posting devotions on Facebook, and witnessing to needy souls.

God uses her to reach people who would be turned off by the shy, sweet sister of God.

"God didn't make a mistake when He made you. You need to see yourself as God sees you." Joel Osteen

We are God's people. Like sheep, we follow Christ. The next time we find ourselves in the throes of a binge, with a bloated stomach and foggy mind, thank God for not making a mistake. Pray for Him to break through the muddy vision, and take over your life. You aren't a mistake. You're a miracle.

Prayer: Use me where I am to further Your kingdom.

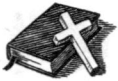

December 2

Praise God and Pass the Biscuits

Enter into his gates with thanksgiving, and into his courts with praise, be thankful unto him, and bless his name. For the Lord is good; his mercy is everlasting and his truth endureth to all generations. Psalms 100:4,5

No food is bad or off limits. When we turn our eating over to God, food loosens its hold. Praise, not *poor me,* captures our focus.

This time of year brings the hundredth Psalm to remembrance. The Lord is good. His mercy never stops. His truth prevails to our children and grandchildren. Bless Him for who He is. Awake with thankfulness on our tongues.

A heart that lingers on the Lord lacks room to ponder pie. A mind stayed on Christ copes better with calamity. This time of year produces food focus. Those able to control their eating at other times of the year get a taste of what compulsive overeaters deal with daily. At Thanksgiving, we must select the superior and concentrate on Christ.

Maintain thanks
Lift praise every day
Forever indebted
Addiction allayed

Praise, and not food
Gratitude, but not gravy
A prayerful attitude
Will soak my mind daily

Prayer: I live with unlimited gratitude to the Lord.

336

December 3

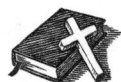

Plug Into the Power Source

But you shall receive power (ability, efficiency, and might) when the Holy Spirit has come upon you and you shall be My witnesses in Jerusalem and all Judea and Samaria and to the ends (the very bounds) of the earth. Acts 1:8 TAB

I have an extra refrigerator in my garage that holds drinks and large or extra foods. Like most refrigerators, it has a light bulb to brighten the inside, so I can make out what's in the back or bottom. A few days ago, I opened the door, but the inside remained dark. I checked everything. The cord was plugged into the wall. The fuse box indicated power pulsed to that plug. I opened the door again. Light flickered on and back off again. I caught hold the bulb and screwed it tighter. Light flooded the box with constant illumination.

The bulb maintained the capacity to light. Power flowed to the plugs, and from the plug to the appliance. Then, what was the problem? The bulb relaxed its connection to the power source. It held light, but wavered with the least touch.

We're like that bulb. God may have saved us. At some point, the Holy Spirit might've come to reside in our hearts. But God will not force His power on us. God expects us to keep the conduit free of obstruction. It's up to us to keep our power-finders tight into the power-giving socket.

When we grow lax in our time with God, or when we start relying on our own abilities to fight the food demon, God's power can't reach us. Like the light bulb in my refrigerator, we may have days or hours of power, but the looseness with which we handle our connection with the Lord can break down with the slightest impediment.

Prayer: Help me keep my connection tight in the grip of the powerful God.

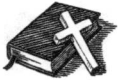

December 4

Rain Down

Your own soul is nourished when you are kind; it is destroyed when you are cruel. Proverbs 11:17

My husband and I gazed across our back yard. A strip of dark green grass stood two inches taller than the rest of the yard that was barely green.

"Obviously, you didn't finish the mowing," I said.

"I mowed it all three days ago." Charles dipped his chin. A smirk twitched at the corner of his mouth. "But I forgot and left the soaker hose going all night on that spot."

My brow furrowed. "Did you fertilize?"

"I fertilized all of it, but that's the only spot that got watered." He was grinning now.

Suddenly, it struck me how that grass reminded me of our souls. We can listen to the sermon on Sunday but, if we don't apply it to our lives with a Holy Spirit watering, the effect is minimal.

One spot at the very tip of our back yard remained brown. My husband said that when he set the sprinkler, the water never quite reached that spot. He had to take a hose and stand in the heat to let water run onto it. He didn't often do that, so the grass withered.

So, too, if we fail to shine God's light on our food choices and activity selections, that corner of our life does nothing to further our walk with Christ. Nourishment makes us willing witnesses. Missing out on Holy Spirit power tears down our testimony.

Prayer: Nourish me today, and water it with Holy Spirit rain.

December 5

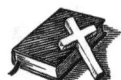

Like New

By abolishing in His (own crucified) flesh the enmity (caused by) the Law with its decrees and ordinances (which He annulled); that He from the two might create in Himself one new man (one new quality of humanity out of the two), so making peace.
Ephesians 2:15 TAB

I made a bed on the floor of our den out of old quilts. My grandsons would sleep there during the holidays. My mother-in-law's wrinkled hands picked up one of the quilts. "Ooh, I love this pattern. I haven't seen it for years."

I told her that indeed it was the quilt I played on as a child. "I've always loved it, but now it's all ripped and torn. I use it only on the floor or outside for a picnic."

"No, no, this is too fine for that," she said. "I'll fix it."

She asked permission to take home my old quilt and mend it. I agreed, but I admit that I didn't expect much improvement. The poor thing had seen too much wear to be of further use.

However, Granny is a master at quilting and sewing.

The next time we visited her she gave me the *new,* old quilt. My eyes lit with excitement. New material brightened the older part. Sparkling satin bound the edges. No torn places marred the cover. Memories of my childhood were sparked. I brought home the quilt. Since it matched my guest room bedspread, I folded it at the end of the bed like a decoration. The room was revived. Who could know?

In the verse above, the missionary, Paul, talks of uniting Christian Jews and Gentiles. Since both loved Jesus, peace mended the breach. Our lives can be torn and messy from overeating, emotional outbursts, and silent seething, but the Lord can mend our lives and make them new.

Prayer: Today, fix all my ripped edges and twisted parts.

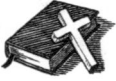

December 6

WWJD

Follow God's example in everything you do as a much-loved child imitates his father. Ephesians 5:1 Life Recovery Bible

Each year, our church hosts the men from Life Challenge of Dallas. Men of all ages sing and testify about God's work in their lives while they live and work in this program. There, each seeks deliverance from drug and alcohol addictions. Yesterday, one man's testimony stuck in my mind as something we all need to remember from time to time.

After spending nearly two years in this drug rehabilitation program, this man faced the time of re-entering normal life. He said he worried over what he should do and where he should live, but that morning, he searched his Bible for the answer. God led him to the verse above. His version read more like, "Just follow Jesus wherever He goes."

A few years ago, it became popular to wear a bracelet or a T-shirt that asked the question: "What would Jesus do?" Many people wore that as with any fad without thinking about what it said. Still, the verse above that helped that Christian ex-drug addict still resonates in my mind today as I write this devotion.

Who of us has not seen a young boy attempt to do exactly what his daddy did, whether it was drive a racecar or hammer a nail? Christianity boils down to that simple principle.

When we eat, we should follow Christ. How would we feel if Jesus sat at the dinner table with us, or in an easy chair with a bag of Reese's candy, or stood beside us as we ate from the gallon container of ice cream?

"WWJD"?

Prayer: Keep my eyes stayed on Your lead today.

December 7

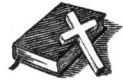

No Mighty Food

No weapon that is formed against thee shall prosper; and every tongue that shall rise against thee in judgment thou shalt condemn... Isaiah 54:17

Food never gained supremacy over my husband. Through the years, he remained slender. However, these last few years, his metabolism slowed, medicines he took interfered with weight maintenance, and his activity isn't as much as it used to be.

For the first time in his life, he must watch what he eats. Mostly, that's not a problem. He's not a big-time snacker, but he can't leave his ice cream alone, and he can't do without butter.

His weight won't stay down because of those two foods.

In weight loss circles, we call those trigger foods. We each have something that tempts us and trips us more often than others. Foods fall into two categories: sweet or salty, chips or cake. I've started lots of diets with the idea that I could give up candy and donuts for awhile, but I couldn't give them up forever. Yes, my problem is sweets.

God says no weapon can prosper against His children. Nothing can befall the child of God that can overcome us unless we allow it.

No difficult circumstance.

No illness that causes a sedentary lifestyle.

No busy lifestyle where eating out is required.

And no mighty food.

Until I released my hold on candy and donuts, God couldn't protect me from them. When we say, "Okay, I give them up for You," the Lord wins and so do we.

Prayer: I give up my trigger food today and each day with Your help.

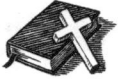

December 8

Stewardship

His lord said unto him, Well done, thou good and faithful servant; thou hast been faithful over a few things, I will make thee ruler over many things; enter thou into the job of thy lord.
Matthew 25;21

Shut in with three young children, I felt my sanity slip. Life went on without me while I sat at home building sofa forts and reciting nursery rhymes.

Money burned a hole in my pocket, but I had no car to go to the store. I dreamed of powdered donuts and Baby Ruth candy bars. I knew I'd feel better if I could just get something good to eat. I needed *Me* time. For lunch, I fixed mashed potatoes and macaroni and cheese; two of my daughter's favorites. I heated green beans to assuage my guilt at not having vegetables. I spent my grocery budget on the steak to serve my husband that night. Still, my billfold held a twenty, and a convenience store stood on the highway less than a mile away.

"Let's take a walk," I told my girls, convincing myself I was doing this for my children. They could buy a treat, and I could exercise.

How many times do compulsive overeaters overspend their resources and lie to themselves about the true purpose? God made us stewards over our family incomes, whether it comes from us, our mates, or a combined effort. Junk food empties our pockets and sedates our minds.

Are we being good stewards of our money, time, energy? Are we using our minds to improve ourselves or tear down our effectiveness?

Prayer: Remind me that what I have is given by You and deserves good stewardship from me.

December 9

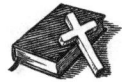

A Full Moon

Where were you when I laid the foundations of the earth? Tell me, if you know so much. Do you know how its dimensions were determined and who did the surveying?
Job 38:4,5 Life Recovery Bible

A full moon lit up the summer sky as bright as a cloudy day. We sat outside and watched with wonder at God's majesty on display. After much belly-aching and bad counsel from friends, Job cried out to God for mercy. God answered with rare words that told us something of creation.

Our human mind can't begin to understand the speed of light zipping across the universe. To us, the moon looks constant, close, and incredible. This month God is giving us two full moons; a bonus of stunning scenes.

In the scope of understanding a full moon, an overeating compulsion appears easy to manage. It is for the Lord. The next time we feel beaten up and ready to quit, remember the moon is but a mound of debris, yet reflects the light shined against its surface and thereby gives beauty to all on earth.

T hank
H eaven for the
A wesome
N ewness of the
K ing

Prayer: Shine on me today, so that I might reflect your wonder.

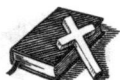

December 10

Think Outside the Box

As for God, his way is perfect; the word of the Lord is tried: he is a buckler to all them that trust in him. 2 Samuel 22:31

A few years ago, Taco Bell put out a new slogan: "Think outside the box." Fast food addicts, who headed to such places as McDonalds and Burger King to get hamburgers, now stopped for tacos. The slogan worked. The taco business grew and surpassed many hamburger places.

Controlling, compulsive individuals plan their days in precision format. We begin with a to-do list and mark off our objectives. We allow little room for God to work. We demand our own way and sulk over interruptions.

I'm guilty as charged.

Are you innocent?

When it comes to losing weight, we trust in tried and true methods. We plot our graphs, we write down our food expectations, we expect a loss to reward our efforts.

God's plans are not ours. God provides losses on His timetable and in His way. All our frustration and anger over a friend's stopping by with donuts, or weeks of no weight loss could be God's idea of "thinking outside the box." God's way is perfect. We must keep our minds centered on the main thing, and the main thing isn't weight loss. The most important thing is to follow God's will.

Today, at the top of our lists, number one priority, we must write down, FOLLOW WHERE GOD LEADS, regardless of how *different* or *anti-weight-loss* it appears.

Prayer: Fix my mind on following You today, not on losing or maintaining weight.

December 11

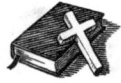

Fill Her Up

Let him kiss me with the kisses of his mouth; for thy love is better than wine. Song of Solomon 1:2

He gazed at her with softened blue-gray eyes. He moved closer so that his expelled air warmed her waiting lips. "I love you."

Her breath caught. Her legs threatened to buckle. She grabbed the arm for support. His handsome face would linger in her mind long after he turned from her. "How I've longed to hear those words." A strand of hair fell across her face.

Gentle fingers brushed her cheek and pulled back her hair. "And . . . ?"

"Your love fills my heart and soul to overflowing."

His strong hands sought the small of her back and drew her to him, so that his heart kept rhythm with hers.

I write Christian romance. No greater love story exists than the one between Jesus and His bride.

My father owned service stations back in the sixties and seventies before self-serve became popular. A customer would pull in and tell him, "Fill her up," meaning fill their gas tank to the brim with gasoline.

Giving up your addiction or compulsion or cleansing your mind from resentment and anger isn't enough. Jesus tells us that when a demon is cast out, he finds the vessel still empty and goes to get seven more demons and reenters. When you surrender to God, ask him to "fill her up" with His love.

Fall in love with Jesus.

Prayer: Keep love overflowing in my heart and mind, so that You become the lover of my soul.

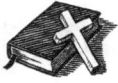

December 12

Hell or Heaven

The sorrows of hell compassed me about; the snares of death prevented me. Psalms 18:5

Helplessness	Destruction
Hopelessness	Defilement
Hell	Death
Emptiness	Exiled
Enslavement	

No words can adequately describe a compulsive overeater in the throes of the disease.

Frustrated at trying to make me feel better, my husband beseeched me to want to live for my family that loved me.

I couldn't see what he saw. My view was warped, my mind was clouded. To me, my family would be better off if I died. My husband could stop dealing with my depressive tirades. My children wouldn't have to hear my emotional outbursts. Their lives would improve. They would even get money from my life insurance. To me, it was a clear choice.

God gives us new words.

Life	Peace
Love	Hope
Faith	Mercy
Healing	Grace
Joy	Heaven

Remember God's words. They'll pull a compulsive overeater or addict from hell. Use your favorite word daily.

Prayer: Remind me of Your words when I need them.

December 13

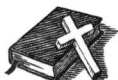

What About Other People?

And be ye kind, one to another, tenderhearted, forgiving one another, even as God for Christ's sake hath forgiven you.
Ephesians 4:32

How long has it been since you read the golden rule? How long since you thought about others?

Compulsive or addictive personalities dwell on themselves way too much. We are a selfish bunch. It's all about us and how rough we have it.

At one time, I had a coworker who complained daily. It wasn't that she didn't have problems. She had legitimate difficulties: poor health, a drug-addicted son, financial trouble. I fought depression because of the burdens of her negativity. But there was one thing that was good about it—I realized how blessed I was. So every time I got depressed from listening to her, I turned it into counting my blessings.

One surefire cure to the doldrums is helping someone else. Practice the golden rule, and we get our minds off ourselves. A recent magazine presented fifty tips on ways to be kind. Make your own list. What could you do to help someone just to be kind, maybe something no one would know about but us? While we think of this, we don't think of food.

The Christmas season is a superb time to show God's love to others.

"We make a living by what we get. We make a life by what we give." Winston Churchill

Prayer: Direct my focus today to someone where I can show kindness.

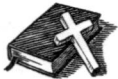

December 14

Anger Ends in Death

A wise man feareth, and departeth from evil, but the fool rageth, and is confident. He that is soon angry dealeth foolishly; and a man of wicked devices is hated. Proverbs 14:16,17

Anger is a small seed
That grows in fertile minds
Dwelling in proportion
To thoughts that we let bind.

It ties us up in knots
Confounds all our emotion,
It starts a process in us
Of steady, sad erosion.
                    By Janet K. Brown

Anger captures its prisoners and refuses to let them go. Nothing hurts us more. We can stuff in our mouths more food than we can eat in a lifetime, and that will not destroy the poison of anger permeating our systems. It ties the ropes around us tighter until there's no escape except through God's healing strength. Left to simmer, non-released anger kills its victims as surely as if we thrust knives into our hearts.

Anger.
I release you now.
I cannot hold onto you
Else you cause my death.
                    By Janet K. Brown

Prayer: Teach me to let anger go. Heal me, Lord.

December 15

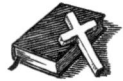

Sizzle

Then laid they their hands on them, and they received the Holy Ghost. Acts 8:17

Streaks of lightning bolted from the sky around my car. My grip on the steering wheel tightened. My heart beat faster. I felt a little sizzle of lightning though, thankfully, without injury.

My husband and I toured the Mesa Verde National Park near Durango, Colorado. What an interesting place that is. Rain clouds built up in the west but nothing looked so bad as to bring alarm. I leaned over a precipice to look down into the ruins of a home built by the ancients. Suddenly, my hair tingled, my skin felt on fire, and the tree beside me shot fire. My legs were glued to the ground. I couldn't move. My husband grabbed my hand and pulled me away from the place. We left, but I never forgot that experience.

I will never forget another experience. The Holy Spirit touched me. I felt His power surge through my heart and mind. Nothing looked the same after the sizzle from the Holy Ghost. I looked at things from a different point of view. I acted with more boldness. I witnessed more easily.

Boredom leads compulsive overeaters to food. We search for excitement, as the country song goes, in all the wrong places. The sugary taste of a cream-filled donut disappears after the morsel slides down your throat. The spicy flavor of pepperoni pizza can satisfy hunger, but that's all it can do. Only the Holy Spirit can quench the desire for joy in our lives.

If you're looking for something exciting, ask God for His sizzle.

Prayer: Satisfy my heart with the happiness that comes only from You.

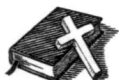

December 16

Controller

Don't drink too much wine, for many evils lie along that path; be filled instead with the Holy Spirit and controlled by him.
Ephesians 5:18 Life Recovery Bible

My grandson sat in front of his X-Box, the controller in his hand. "Come on, Mimi. I've got two controllers. You can fight me."

That's how I found out I'm not too good with X-Box controllers. My character didn't seem to do what I was trying to get him to do, while my grandson's whipped past every hindrance.

How like real life, that is. We slave to make all the parts of our life balance out and excel, but our "man" (or woman) just won't do what we want them to do. We turn to crutches to soothe the hurt. Some drink too much wine or reach for the harder liquor. Some go for gambling, indulgent shopping or, like some of us, excess food.

"In your heart of hearts, ask yourself, What do I really want in my life? Do I want a body to rival the latest cover on my favorite magazine, or do I want happiness and a deep sense of inner joy?" From *The Spiritual Path to Weight Loss* by Gregory L. Jantz, Ph.D.

Like with video games, the proper controller is required to make it work. Who's in control of your man?

Prayer: Fill me and control me, today.

December 17

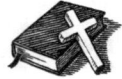

Elephants

That he would grant you, according to the riches of his glory, to be strengthened with might by his Spirit in the inner man.
Ephesians 3:16

Elephants fascinate us. They're the largest land-bound mammal. At birth, they weigh an average of 230 pounds and grow to thousands of pounds at maturity. The distinguishing characteristic is the trunk. It's so sensitive it can pick up a single blade of grass, yet so strong, it can rip off tree branches. The adult elephant has no natural predators. Its loud trumpeting sound intimidates men and beasts.

Asian countries consider the elephant a symbol of wisdom. Because of their extreme memory and intelligence, men can train an elephant despite their overpowering size by chaining them when they're small and using prods and picks to make them obey commands. The elephant never forgets the effect of the torture, and always believes that the stake in the ground will restrict them even when they grow big enough to attack their capturers.

Compulsive overeaters can identify with elephants. We fear failure and believe in our inability to overcome the compulsion because of the memory of our defeats. Even after periods of success, our minds bring forth our failures. Our mouths water, and we succumb to expected temptation, not realizing that, all the time, we've grown in strength. Our inner man is powerful because of God's Spirit in us.

Let's forget the failures of the past. Remember, the Spirit enlarges our capacity for victory.

Prayer: Grant me Your strength and the riches of Your glory.

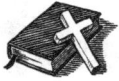

December 18

Sponsor Me

Because of and through the heart of tender mercy and loving-kindness of our God, a Light from on high will dawn upon us and visit (us). To shine upon and give light to those who sit in darkness and in the shadow of death to direct and guide our feet in a straight line into the way of peace. Luke 1:78,79 TAB

In a twelve step program such as Overeaters Anonymous, a new person wanders in from the darkness and the shadow of binge-driven misery. In my first meeting, my jaw dropped at the familiar strains. One person after another told *my* story, although in their unique voice. Tears started to stream my face. My heart melted like an ice cube in ninety-degree sunshine.

The first thing the group advises you to do is get a sponsor; that's a person who's walked where you walked and can advise you what steps to take. That person makes themselves available day or night to an emergency call.

The twelve-step programs use members to help other members. The wisdom of that idea came from Jesus, who chose twelve disciples to take the message to hurting people.

When we start the path toward weight loss and a healing from overeating compulsion, we ask Jesus to be our sponsor. He underwent every temptation known to man without sin. He understands. He can light our feet and direct our food plans.

Still, Jesus ordains we help each other. As God leads you, consider guiding others with that God-given insight. Others helped us on our way. A wonderful man stared a Christian Weight Controllers group in our church, and pulled me out of the darkness. I praise God for sending him and his wife my way. I pray God use me as sponsor to others wherever I meet them.

Prayer: Help me cling to Jesus as my sponsor, and use me as sponsor to direct others to You.

December 19

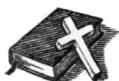

Depression

When thou passest through the waters, I will be there, and through the rivers, they shall not overflow thee; when thou walkest through the fire, thou shalt not be burned; neither shall the flame kindle upon thee. Isaiah 43:2

This time of year plagues many, especially those who've lost loved ones or are separated from them. It also hurts those from dysfunctional families who hate Christmas scenes of mom, dad, and children around the tree. Satan's cruel plan is to desires to destroy this season of peace and good will or, at least, ruin it for many. Jesus understands betrayal and disappointment.

Trampled Violets

Trampled underneath
By uncaring feet
Bruised and crushed
The petals scattered
Violets in first blush
Of bloom.
Disillusioned, hurt
By cruel words
Stomped and torn
The child succumbs
To hatred of his known
Small world.
Mocked and spit upon
By His own
Stabbed and slapped
His hands were pierced
His words were spoken
Forgive.   By Janet K. Brown

Prayer: I cling to You, the healer of depression.

353

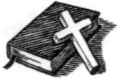

December 20

It's God's Command

For if ye forgive men their trespasses, your heavenly Father will also forgive you; But if ye forgive not men their trespasses, neither will your Father forgive your trespasses.
Matthew 6:14, 15

Some offenses are hard to forgive. Those hurts directed toward us when we were children lay like open wounds, oozing infection. Years of psychotherapy can't provide enough ointment to apply as a balm.

God forgives us. We must forgive others. When we let go the anger and resentment that we hold for wrongs perpetrated on us, God frees us to love and laugh and be free.

"There is a thin line that separates laughter and pain, comedy and tragedy, humor and hurt." Erma Bombeck

In Christianity, forgiveness isn't an option. If we are to live, we must yield all ire.

The madder I get, the more I eat, the more I yell or pout, and the more I dive into other compulsive behaviors.

FORGIVE
or
DIE

Prayer: Lord, help me daily forgive, so that I'm free to receive Your touch.

December 21

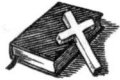

Hold Me Upright

The spirit of the Lord God is upon me; because the Lord hath anointed me to preach good tidings unto the meek; he hath sent me to bind up the brokenhearted, to proclaim liberty to the captives, and the opening of the prison to them that are bound; Isaiah 61:1

Yesterday, the devil tripped me. I lay flat on the ground, feeling helpless and without worth. I think God allowed it. While on the ground, I looked up to Him. I needed a little reminder that it's all about Him. I've been a little puffed up and thought I was hot stuff because I got my first book published. God decided I needed a reminder of how important I was.

I wish I could draw. I would illustrate a prone figure with God's powerful arm reaching down to pick me off the cold ground. His muscles ripple. My scrawny body is limp in his hand.

God, You are so good. I magnify Your name.

Glory and power and honor are Yours.

Let me decrease, so that You might increase.

Here I am writing devotions about my healing from compulsive overeating, and I fall to my knees with chocolate smeared around my mouth and dribbling off my chin. I have as much strength as the mosquito I just squashed between my hands.

God gives the healing. Only God keeps me upright.

In a day where desserts tempt, and stress is pushing us to rush and finish the hundreds of things to be done before Christmas, walk with us. Don't let go of our hand.

Prayer: Thanks for the reminder to look to You before life overwhelms me.

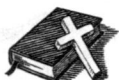

December 22

Little Is Much

He that is faithful in that which is least is faithful also in much;
Luke 16:10

God is the best mathematician I know.
He understands how to multiply.
He never wastes His resources, so
Bring the vessels and don't ask why.
    Phoebe was a plain little lady
    Who took Paul's letter to Rome
    We'll not know the result of that trip
    Till we get eternally home.
Jesus watched the gate of the temple
As the widow dropped in her mite.
He knew God would expand it.
It was stupendous in His sight.
    Priscilla and Aquila, humble tentmakers
    Welcomed Paul into their home.
    God used their love and influence
    Through Paul, everywhere that he roamed.
Who's to say that Na-aman
Would've received healing at that hour
Had not his wife's servant girl
Told of God's healing power?
    Israel's spies would've been killed
    But for a sinner named Rahab.
    God used her act of kindness
    And added to her heavenly tab.
It seems God can use anyone
Any problem or personality.
The only requirement is yielding
With submission and loyalty. (Poem continued tomorrow)

Prayer: Help me to be the little in Your hand, today.

December 23

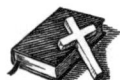

It Doesn't Take a Mighty Person

Philip answered him, two hundred pennyworth of bread is not suf-
ficient for them, that every one of them may take a little. John 6:7

As Philip discovered in the verse above, Jesus changes things.
In His hands, small, insignificant seeds of obedience flourish and
a small amount of bread feeds thousands.

Dorcas gave her talent for sewing.
Lydia, her fine large home.
They served Christ in their home towns
But God made their small deeds known.
    Yes, though we serve Him in secret,
    He can still use the vessel we give.
    He can turn that small cup of water
    To a source so that others might live.
The widow in Elijah's day
Gave the man of God to eat.
Then the meal and oil were multiplied.
Only God could do that feat.
    God used Jochabed and a princess
    To save Moses to lead a nation.
    He used a mother and grandmother
    To train Timothy against temptation.
God used many examples and stories
He fed multitudes fish and bread
To show us multiplication power,
If we but do what He says.
    But me, I have little to offer
    Though I follow Jesus' command
    But even little can be much
    When put into Jesus' hand.   By Janet K. Brown

Prayer: Heal my compulsion and use me today.

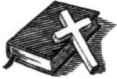

December 24

Too Much Time with Loved Ones

Love endures long and is patient and kind; love never is envious nor boils over with jealousy, is not boastful or vainglorious, does not display itself haughtily. 1 Corinthians 13:4 TAB

I lost my mother nineteen years ago. The first Christmas without her, I grieved for her presence. I still miss her every day. The truth was that nearly every visit, she would hurt my feelings. She loved me and never came to our house with that intent. However, during her visit, we would always clash.

Since she was a neat nut, I would spend days cleaning house before she arrived, but she set about to "get some spots I didn't have time to clean." I didn't show much patience or kindness and took it as an insult to my housecleaning. Her five-feet viewed my two hundred fifty pounds as an indictment on her, so she couldn't help but pointing out that I ought to eat less.

Christmas brings families together. Sometimes we end up with hurt feelings, disappointments, or full-scale verbal battles. Though we're excited to see them and wouldn't dream of leaving them out, many of us have a mom, an Aunt Mildred, or Uncle Fred, who always makes us feel small.

Look at what that verse mentions we should do:
- Endure it/let it go.
- Be patient.
- Be kind.
- Don't envy.
- Don't compare.
- Don't boast.
- Don't think of yourself more highly than others.

I might add an extra one. Don't allow hurtful words to make you overeat.

Prayer: This Christmas, remind me of your mercy and help me show grace even to that loved one that pulls my chain.

December 25

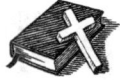

Prince of Peace

For unto us a child is born, unto us a son is given; and the government shall be upon his shoulder and his name shall be called Wonderful, Counselor, the mighty God, The everlasting Father, the Prince of Peace. Isaiah 9:6

MERRY CHRISTMAS ✝ MERRY CHRISTMAS ✝ MERRY CHRISTMAS

This day will be celebrated across the world in different ways. Some will feast with families. Others grieve alone. However this day finds us, one thing is sure.

This day, this season, brings challenges for the compulsive overeater.

Today, more food abounds, even to the poor, due to the generosity of churches or food banks. More depression plagues people because we've built up this season to be the perfect situation. It rarely works out quite that way. Most people seek family and leave out those alone. Even Christian congregations reach out in the days before Christmas, but not on the actual day. Soup kitchens and missions fill with the lonely and hurting. Some in the midst of family feel left out and adrift.

As you read your devotion this day, consider this. We won't gain a lot of weight over one day of indulgence. It's making the month of December a feasting celebration that loads pounds on everyone. A compulsive overeater, though not alone at this time in eating too much, is more at risk for not being able to stop and change course afterward.

Let us use this day to praise the Lord for days of healing and for any weight already lost. Let's be grateful for healthy food to eat and the ability to move without extra pounds. Concentrate on what you have, not what you've lost.

Prayer: Lord, remind me today of how blessed we are to have You.

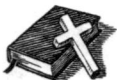

December 26

Stuffed Stomachs

Ye have heard that it was said by them of old time, THOU SHALT NOT COMMIT ADULTERY; But I say unto you, That whosover looketh on a woman to lust after her hath committed adultery with her already in his heart. Matthew 5:27,28

Jesus gave several references like this that tells us our minds sin before we commit the act. What does that say about what we feed our minds?

"In effect, the subconscious mind is like a battery. From it, you can obtain tremendous surges of mental and spiritual energy which often transmute themselves into practical vitality. These jolts of energy will go to waste if we permit them to be short-circuited." *Success Through a Positive Mental Attitude* by Napoleon Hill and W. Clement Stone

My husband and I used to sell Amway products. We attended endless motivational conferences and kept an uplifting CD playing all the time. One thing we were warned about was to not engage in "stinking thinking."

The devil can't read our minds, but he can hear our words. When we speak negatives such as "I'm a fat slob," or "I'll never lose weight, or "I'm too weak," we reinforce what our minds think and get that thought out for the devil to replay for us.

If, on this day after Christmas, you have leftover pie that tempts you, bless a neighbor or someone in your church with a piece, send it home with a family member, or throw it in the waste can—not on your body's bulging waist. If you're healthy, dwell on doing something active today, whether you still have company or not. Get up early to enjoy quiet time with the Lord before the day gets hectic. Stuff your mind with good stuff, not your stomach.

Prayer: Fill my mind with hope as I think on You.

December 27

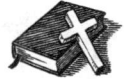

Let Go

There is a saying, Love your friends and hate your enemies.
But I say; Love your enemies! Pray for those who persecute you.
Matthew 5:43,44 Life Recovery Bible

In Overeaters Anonymous, a saying reverberates around the meetings. "Let go and let God." A local hospital for the mentally challenged gives out this list of "let go" definitions.

- To let go does not mean to stop caring, it means I can't do it for someone else.
- To let go is not to cut myself off, it's the realization I can't control another.
- To let go is to admit powerlessness, which means the outcome is not in my hands.
- To let go is not to fix, but to support.
- To let go is not to judge, but to allow another to be human.
- To let go is not to be protective, it's to permit another to face reality.
- To let go is not to deny, but to accept.
- To let go is not to nag, scold, or argue, but instead to search out my own shortcomings and correct them.
- To let go is not to adjust everything to my desires but to take each day as it comes, and cherish myself in that.
- To let go is to not criticize and regulate anybody but to try to become what I dream I can be.
- To let go is not to regret the past, but to grow and live for the future.
- To let go is to fear less and love more.
- To let go is to not enable, but to allow learning from natural consequences.
- To let go is not to try to change or blame another, it's to make the most of myself.
- To let go is not to care for, but to care about.

Prayer: Help me to let go and let God, today.

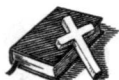

December 28

Persistence of Salmon

For thou are my lamp, O Lord; and the Lord will lighten my darkness. For by thee I have run through a troop; by my God have I leaped over a wall. 2 Samuel 22:29,30

While visiting our daughter and son-in-law in Colorado, we drove to Estes Park. What a beautiful place that is. As we walked along the river, we saw thousands of salmon seeking to jump to the top of a waterfall.

Before they lay their eggs, salmon head upstream to reach their own hatching place, regardless of how far they must travel. Some swim thousands of miles. God made the salmon a determined, persistent creature and a lesson for those of us who grow weary.

Another example is the elk. A huge herd took over the golf course and spread along the river. Only one male with a huge rack of horns lay in the middle of the grass surrounded by his harem.

A hundred feet away from the herd stood another male elk. We snapped a picture when he looked at us. He was a bit smaller and younger than the male with the herd. The smaller male awaited his moment when he was strong enough to challenge the other and take over the herd. For now, he laid alone. Again, persistence.

Overcoming a strong compulsion like that of overeating takes a lifetime. Sometimes, we do tire of what we consider the same foods, or of just having to rein in our desires to keep down our weight. The next time, we think of quitting, remember the salmon and the male elk. Persistence may wear on us, but it brings the reward in the end. With God, we can and will make it.

Prayer: Give me strength to go another day.

December 29

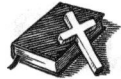

Unequal Results

When the men hired at five o'clock were paid, each received $20. So, when the men hired earlier came to get theirs, they assumed they would receive much more. But they, too, were paid $20. They protested . . . Matthew 20:9-11a, Life Recovery Bible

I attended Weight Watchers with a friend. She's a large, big-boned, young beauty. The pounds seemed to melt off her body. Jealousy teased my thoughts while I tried to build satisfaction for a quarter-pound loss one week, and none the next. Women dieters always envy the men. Their more muscular frames allow more food while they lose three times faster.

We humans like equal results and equal payment. Obviously, that's not a recent opinion. As we read the above parable told by Jesus, we observe the same mindset. A wealthy landowner went into town and hired men to work in his fields for $20 for the day. Thankful to have a job, many went with him under that promise. However, the employer found he needed more helpers, so went he went back and hired an extra crew, also promising them $20. He fulfilled his promises to all the men, but the first group got mad.

Churches fight the same protests. Some who have wor-shiped Christ for years resent new Christians taking over their jobs or filling the church with new ways of doing things.

For my thoughts are not your thoughts, neither are your ways, my ways, saith the Lord. Isaiah 55:8

Resentment and envy will extinguish our healing. We must trust God's direction for our weight loss and/or weight main-tenance. When it seems unfair to us, we must remember God knows best. Our job is to submit to His decisions.

Prayer: I let go my sense of unfairness and give in to Your plan for improvement.

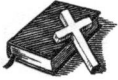

December 30

We Need Each Other

Iron sharpeneth iron so a man sharpeneth the countenance of his friend. Proverbs 27:17.

My husband and I were in a terrible spot financially. I retreated from the known and familiar, wanting to curl up away from the world and ignore our problems. Depression brought me to my knees. I craved more and sweeter foods. While doing only the necessary things for my family, I shut myself within my home and curtailed my contact with people.

One special friend, with wisdom given by God, pestered me to go to lunch with her until I could no longer refuse. She had asked so many times that my excuses sounded lame even to my own ears.

I met her. "I know you're down right now and the last thing you want is for me to pry, but that's exactly what I'm going to do," my friend said. Nothing like honesty to wake up a wayward servant. It was the beginning of my healing years ago.

Solomon advised us of the need for friendship. He says that like iron on iron, we improve each other. My church sponsors "Girlfriends in God," or GIG. Not "ladies fellowship" but girlfriends. All ages meet and visit and work together.

God means us to help each other. Depression and dieting require help. We're most vulnerable when left alone. Our most dangerous time comes when we turn away from the support we need at conquering the compulsion to overeat whether it's through a meeting, a doctor, phone calls or an online chat. Friends keep us accountable, pray for us, and encourage us. Sometimes, a call to a friend can eliminate the gooey temptation calling our names.

Prayer: Thank You for providing me friends or family that metaphorically pull my hands out of the food.

December 31

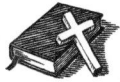

Set Goals and Dream

But God hath revealed them unto us by his Spirit, for the Spirit searcheth all things, yea the deep things of God.
1 Corinthians 2:10

Tomorrow we begin a new year. New Year's resolutions may not work, but setting well-thought-out, written, and prayed-over goals do. It's time to evaluate the illness that tied us in knots. Has God brought an emotional healing during this year? Has He started a new work? Have you hit bottom and you're ready to begin?

Wherever you are on the path, it's time to focus. In the New Year, will it be **God's** Way?

Go through these steps:

D ecide if you're ready to submit to God.

R ead this daily devotion book in the New Year and everything else that will help, especially the Bible.

E nergize through leaving off sugars and fats that drain your vitality.

A dmit your powerlessness and ask God to take over your life.

M entor others as you receive your day-by-day healing.

D iscern God's will daily.

R ecord your progress and reaffirm God's leading.

E at the Word. Make it part of you.

A ssociate with friends that pray and encourage.

M aintain contact with God, regardless of what's going on in your world.

Prayer: I can't. God can. Lead me in the coming year.

ACKNOWLEDGEMENTS

Thank you, Pen-L Publishing for taking a chance on *Divine Dining*. This book brought reality to my dream and God's instruction.

Thank you, Kerry and Lynn McClure, who started the first Christian Weight Controllers in my church nineteen years ago. They were the first to open my eyes to my rebellion against God in the realm of overeating. As teacher, Kerry told me, "Compulsive overeaters possess willpower in abundance. We *will* to eat and do what we choose, not what God offers."

Thank you, Moonine Sue Watson, for reading and critiquing every word of this book, and encouraging me when I faltered.

Thank you, Julia Clark, Christie Coheley, and Cindy Lutter, my three precious daughters who watched me go through years of the highs and lows of compulsive overeating and resistance to God's plan for my life. I love you and your God-sent husbands and children.

Thank you, Charles L. Brown, my sweetheart, husband, and friend for fifty years, who walked with me through depression, disgust, anger, and suicidal thoughts, but never failed to fight for our marriage. His love held fast despite my weight. I love and cherish you.

Most of all, thank you, Lord, for healing me emotionally and setting me on a path I could not have imagined twenty years ago. Eye hath not seen, nor ear heard, what the Lord has in store for us. I love you, Jesus.

BIBLIOGRAPHY

Agnes, Michael, Editor (2003) *Webster's New World Dictionary.* Pocket Books.

Anonymous *(1976) Alcoholics Anonymous*, 3rd edition. Alcoholics Anonymous World Services, Inc.

"Amazing Grace," lyrics, written and performed by Chris Tomlin.

Arterburn, Stephen and David Stoop (1992) The Life Recovery *Bible.* Tyndale House Publisher, Inc.

Danowski, Debbie (2002) *Locked Up for Eating Too Much.* Hazelden Publications.

Hill, Napoleon and W. Clement Stone (1997) *Success Through a Positive Mental Attitude.* Pocket Books.

— (1960) *Think & Grow Rich.* Fawcett-Crest Books.

Maltz, Maxwell (1989) *Psycho-Cybernetics.* Pocket Books.

Maxwell, John (1996) *Partners in Prayer.* Thomas Nelson.

McCutcheon, Marc (1995) *Roget's Super Thesaurus.* Writer's Digest Books.

Meyer, Joyce (2002) *Battlefield of the Mind.* Warner Faith.

Pittman, Bill and Dick B. editors. *Courage to Change.* Hazelden Pittman Archives Press.

Shamblin, Gwen (1997) *The Weigh Down Diet* . Guidepost Editors.

Janet K. Brown

lives in Wichita Falls, Texas, with her husband, Charles. Though she has written most of her adult life, since her retirement as a bookkeeper and medical coder she writes as a second career and as a ministry.

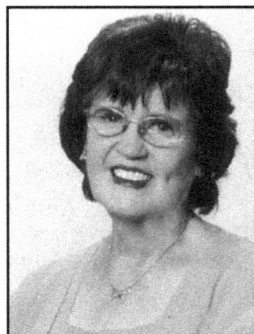

Divine Dining is the author's second book. It encompasses her passion for diet, fitness, and God's Word. Janet released her debut novel, an inspirational young adult, *Victoria and the Ghost,* in July, 2012.

Janet's stories and articles have appeared in *Brio*, *The Gem,*, *Standard*, and *Cross and Quill*. She is a member of American Christian Fiction Writers, Oklahoma Writers Federation, Christian Writers Fellowship Intl. and Romance Writers of America.

Accompanied by her husband, Janet loves to travel with their RV, visit family, and work in their church. After losing ninety-five pounds herself, she's hooked on line dancing and Zumba®.

You can learn more about Janet on her website/blog: http://www.janetkbrown.com. Also, find her on Facebook and Twitter. She'd love to hear from you. E-mail her at Janet.hope@att.net

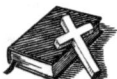

Special Bonus next page!

Special Bonus!

Here's a free sample of Janet's novel, *Worth Her Weight*, available at Pen-L.com, BarnesandNoble.com, Amazon.com in paperback, Kindle and Nook.

How can a woman who gives to everyone but herself accept God's love and healing when she believes she's fat, unworthy, and unfixable?

Happy readers:

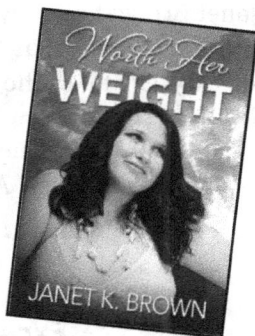

The book was great! And true to the way a food addict deals with their struggles. I know first-hand. Love the book.
~ DeeLynn Lopez, Program Director of Behavioral Health Group and Co-leader for Celebrate Recovery

In her women's fiction work, Worth Her Weight, author Janet K. Brown carries her readers on Lacey's journey of struggle, failure, heartbreak and redemption. She explores her character's food addiction with the knowledge of someone who has taken on the challenge herself and won. Fear, low self-esteem, and faith are well defined throughout the story.

The novel delivers a Christian message for victims of food addiction without being preachy. The book also chronicles the often dependent, demanding attitude of an elderly parent toward a child in the role of caregiver.

I would recommend this novel to any reader who enjoys books that deal with real life issues and includes the element of sweet romance told from a Christian worldview.
~ Patti Shene

A wonderful story! Lacey Chandler is like many of us–overweight, unhealthy and trying to juggle too many demands. Janet Brown really gets into the emotions and thoughts of her characters. The story is well-thought out and believable with a satisfying ending.

~ Marla Jones

Janet Brown has truly written her heart into *Worth Her Weight*. Exposing areas that those struggling with food addiction and obesity, she takes the reader into the heart of her character and leads the reader through the journey to redemption. A good read, highly recommended.

~ Bonnie Lanthripe, Author of *The Ringleader*

Excerpt from Chapter 14

Without a word, Mom held out a letter to Lacey.

A cold shiver shook her—the same foreboding she had sensed in the morning. "What's this?"

Her mother shrugged. "Came in today's mail."

Lacey opened it, her Mom watching as she read.

She threw the paper across the room. It bounced halfway back to her. "Well, if that doesn't take the cake." She paced, her heels clicking on the scratched and scarred kitchen tiles. The noise level grew louder when she snatched plates from the cabinet and dropped them to the table.

"Save the dishes." Mom's tone was dry, with no humor.

Something like a growl escaped Lacey's lips. "Katie makes the messes. Lacey cleans them up. Isn't that right, Mom?" She crossed her arms over her chest and glared at her mother. "Did you know about this?" Her fingers began drumming on her opposite forearm. Her jaw got so tight, it hurt.

Her mother shook her head. She glanced at Rachel.

The anger was difficult for Lacey to swallow, but she tried. "Sweetie, go wash your hands before we eat."

The child scooted a chair toward the sink.

Lacey halted her. "Go to the bathroom and use the stool there." Her voice shook from her effort at control.

Rachel looked at the pizza with longing, but she obeyed.

The pepperoni and mozzarella aroma permeated the house. Nausea churned in Lacey's stomach despite how good it smelled.

"Has Katie gone?" Mom asked with a soft tone.

In contrast, Lacey nearly yelled. "Of course, she has!"

The lines in Mom's face seemed to deepen. Her skin paled. Lacey was sure the cane was the only thing that kept Mom from falling as she coped with the pain inflicted by her favorite daughter.

The fight had gone out of Lacey. Her knees wobbled. She eased into a chair and nodded. "She wants me to have custody of Rachel. She doesn't even want her own daughter, Mom. What kind of woman walks away from her flesh and blood?"

A whimper came from the living room.

Heat rushed up Lacey's neck. She jumped up and ran, wishing she could erase her careless words.

Rachel curled into a ball on the sofa, her right thumb inserted firmly in her mouth.

"Aunt Lacey's sorry. I didn't mean what I said."

Rachel sucked harder, pulling it out momentarily to speak. "Is my mama coming to get me today?"

"No, sweetheart, not today. Maybe another day." She patted her niece's bare legs.

The sucking sound grew louder. Lacey sat on the floor patting and wondering what to say or do. A clap of thunder reminded her of the unsettled clouds. "I need to go close my car windows. I'll be right back."

She ran outside, started the car, and raised her driver's side window. Just as she got back inside, the downpour had begun.

Mom still sat at the kitchen table, her head in her hands. She rose, grabbing her cane. Red puffy eyes alerted Lacey to her mother's tears, something that seldom happened.

Compassion knocked at Lacey's heart, but she locked it out, when she realized the tears were all for Katie.

Lacey sat on the floor beside Rachel. "You ready for some pizza?" Lacey wanted kids one day, but she wanted her own with a husband by her side. She couldn't attract a man, but now she had a child to raise.

Mom plopped into her recliner. "Do you think food will fix everything?"

"Works for me." Lacey tried a teasing note. "Whenever things go wrong, food makes it better." She huffed at Mom and grimaced. "Didn't you know that?" Good thing she hadn't planned on the cruise. She crunched up the pamphlet and threw it in the trash along with a few other dreams. She'd stay fat and lonely.

What was she going to do with a four-year-old?

More Great Reads
at
Pen-L.com

www.ingramcontent.com/pod-product-compliance
Lightning Source LLC
Chambersburg PA
CBHW072107270326
41931CB00010B/1482